The differences between a man's and a woman's biochemistry are so profound that it is a national scandal that we act as if a woman can be healthy on a male diet. From month to month, from birth to the giving of life to the change of life, women face a unique challenge to keep their body chemistry in balance.—Richard A. Kunin, M.D.

MEGA-NUTRITION FOR WOMEN

"Designed to meet the long-neglected special nutritional needs of women—and tailored to every woman's personal biochemistry—Dr. Kunin's revolutionary "Listen to Your Body" diet promotes quick, safe weight loss and permanent weight control . . . provides noncosmetic answers to many common beauty problems . . . even prevents and treats a wide range of female health disorders. Try it. You'll feel the results!"—*Ms. Magazine*

RICHARD A. KUNIN, M.D., is president of the Orthomolecular Medical Society. He is the author of *Mega-Nutrition* and has published and lectured extensively on orthomolecular medicine and psychiatry. He lives and practices in San Francisco, California.

ALSO BY RICHARD A. KUNIN, M.D.

Mega-Nutrition

MEGA-NUTRITION FOR WOMEN

The First Modern Program For Super Health, Beauty, and Weight Control

—Introducing the "Listen to Your Body" Diet

RICHARD A. KUNIN, M.D.

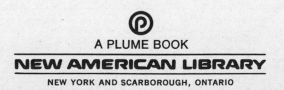

A PLUME BOOK

NEW AMERICAN LIBRARY

NEW YORK AND SCARBOROUGH, ONTARIO

ACKNOWLEDGMENT

For invaluable assistance in the research and writing of this book, I would like to thank Robert E. Burger.

This is an authorized reprint of a hardcover book published by McGraw-Hill Book Company.

Book design by Grace Markman.

Library of Congress Cataloging in Publication Data

Kunin, Richard A.
  Mega-nutrition for women.
  Reprint. Originally published: New York : McGraw-
Hill, 1983
  Bibliography: p.
  Includes index.
  1. Orthomolecular therapy.   2. Reducing diets.
3. Women—Nutrition.   I. Title.
RM235.5.K855   1984   613.2′088042   83-22090
ISBN 0-452-25481-7

SIGNET, SIGNET CLASSIC, MENTOR, PLUME, MERIDIAN and NAL BOOKS are published *in the United States* by New American Library, 1633 Broadway, New York, New York 10019, *in Canada* by The New American Library of Canada Limited, 81 Mack Avenue, Scarborough, Ontario M1L 1M8

First Plume Printing, April, 1984

1 2 3 4 5 6 7 8 9

PRINTED IN THE UNITED STATES OF AMERICA

Contents

For the rest of this century, the American housewife is in a uniquely important role. As never before, *the gift of life* is hers to give or withhold.

— Laurel Robertson, Carol Flinders, Bronwen Godfrey
Laurel's Kitchen

Introduction

A Program for Women—and Intelligent Men

It's time to break with the past. The health care system in this country has been living in the past for nearly a century. It is true that nutrition has had its occasional successes. We're currently going through a strong revival of interest in natural foods, nutrition, and exercise. But we're still bogged down in controversy, frequent extravagant claims, and, perhaps most important, repression of common-sense ideas about well-being by a bureaucratic medical system. As the title of this book indicates, I feel that the best hope for nutrition—and the best *application of* nutrition—is among women. I expect intelligent men to follow their lead.

I'm often asked if "mega-nutrition" isn't just "holistic" medicine. Again, I say the distinction concerns the past. Holistic medicine, for a large part, relies on the past—on meditation, on vegetarianism, on herbalism, on acupuncture, and so on. All of these are time-tested therapeutic modalities. All of them have current application. But the lessons they have for us are already spelled out, for better or for worse. What hasn't been developed to its fullest potential is mega-nutrition. And this is why I call it the medicine of the future. Holistic = past; mega-nutrition = future.

1

I want you to share in the excitement I feel for this. I want you to join me in pursuing the benefits of nutrition beyond the pat answers: a "balanced diet," "getting your RDAs," "the annual physical," and so forth. I want you to see how nutritional research is now so advanced that it needs a new name: "orthomolecular medicine" is one; "mega-nutrition" is another. Perhaps the simplest name is "nutrient therapy." Whatever the name, nutrition will never be the same.

As you might expect, the idea of *diet* has also changed radically. Until nutritional research came of age, dieting was a hit-or-miss affair. It was subject to quackery and fads, to unscientific crash programs that were basically unsafe, to untested gimmicks that were essentially ineffective. Consider the most popular of the recent weight-loss diets:

- The low-carbohydrate diet (Atkins, Drinking Man's diet, Stillman, etc.) has been around since the 1850s, when an English doctor noted its weight-loss potential.
- The Pritikin diet of virtually no fats and high carbohydrates is the diet of necessity of every underdeveloped country in the world.
- The high-fat diet (often the result of going overboard on a low-carbohydrate program) has been time-tested by the Eskimos.
- The Scarsdale diet is one of many short-term low-calorie ideas, often dangerous because nutrients are seldom sufficient.
- The liquid protein (Last Chance) diet turned out to be especially dangerous for the same reason, and has led to many deaths.
- The Cambridge diet combines a drastic calorie reduction with protein powder and a vitamin supplement in powder form.

This last diet deserves some comment, since it comes with a prestigious name attached and makes some pretense at being scientific. It is essentially a liquid protein diet with some of the dangers lessened by the addition of vitamins and minerals. By limiting calories to about á fifth of what most people normally consume, it will result in weight loss. It's better than the Last

Chance diet because it does not ignore such needed minerals as copper and magnesium. But it is seriously low in protein (33 grams a day, even less than the RDA, which itself is arguably low). And the Cambridge diet makes two fundamental assumptions that will inevitably make it useless for many if not most women. First, because it does not supply sufficient essential fatty acids, it will lead to cravings that most people (rightly) will not ignore; it thus almost guarantees *failure*. Second, by assuming that everyone can get by on the exact same ration of protein and carbohydrate, this diet can cause mood changes or serious nutritional deficiencies; this makes it potentially *dangerous*. You can't feed everyone out of a box of powder and hope to meet his or her individual nutrient needs. The basic question in any diet, in fact, is just this: What do *you* need?

This is why I will say, in introducing the Listen to Your Body diet in Chapter Two, that this diet is the first truly *modern* diet. It is the first diet to take all the most recent nutritional research into full account. It is the first diet to take biochemical individuality into account. It is the first diet to teach good nutrition as you use it, the easiest way. It is the first weight-loss diet to help you feel your best and look your best while you shed pounds and inches.

Most fad diets help you lose weight by making you sick— literally sick. But what good is weight loss if you look pale and haggard and if you are irritable and depressed?

Men generally don't undertake a weight-loss program without the fear of a heart attack or other dire warning. Yet the Listen to Your Body diet is for them, too. If my experience is any guide, I think men will take to this program after women have shown how simple and effective it is.

Start with my diet and see if it doesn't do all the things I promise. This is the best introduction to mega-nutrition I can give you. Then see how it gives you a solid foundation for understanding and using all the other nutrient therapies in this book. You and mega-nutrition have a great future together!

Richard A. Kunin, M.D.
San Francisco, California

1
Your Personal Best

The differences between a man's and a woman's biochemistry are so profound that it is a national scandal that we act as if a woman can be healthy on a male diet. The fine print of the Recommended Daily Allowances (RDAs) mentions a few extra requirements for pregnant or lactating women. There is a specialty called gynecology, but one would never guess from those who practice it (males) or from the advances it has made in typical female problems (few) that it is *for* women. From month to month, from birth to the giving of life to the change of life, women face a unique challenge to keep their body chemistry in balance. In recent years, as the dangers of drugs and pollutants in the environment and in food have been uncovered, women of child-bearing age have had to take on new responsibilities. On top of everything else, women are still expected to be the arbiters of diet for most households. And in spite of their natural need for more body fat, they are expected by society to be more weight-conscious.

This book is an attempt to make up for the years of neglect of women's special needs in nutrition. Based on more than two decades of practice in psychiatry and nutritional medicine, my program is a natural way for you to learn to regulate your mental well-being as well as your physical health safely and simply. The mega-nutrition program consists of two adjustments in your diet: (1) the Listen to Your Body diet, or the regulation of the ratio of carbohydrates-fats-protein in your personal regimen, and (2) specific nutrient therapy for your individual medical or psychological problems. My goal is to help you achieve that mixture of the basic food types and nutrients that is *your personal best.*

For several generations of women raised on the catch phrase "balanced diet" and on an industrialized food system, it may be hard to conceive of "personal best" nutrition. But not only are the nutritional requirements of men and women quite different, but the range of needs among women is vast. *You are unique:* in biochemistry this is not a platitude, but a hard reality. I hope to show by case after case how this is so.

But "biochemical individuality" does not mean that the nutrient approach to your special case is necessarily complex or difficult. The wife of a nationally known TV celebrity came to me recently with a complaint that had plagued her for years. She had to get up several times every night for a trip to the bathroom. A weight-conscious dieter, she also had taken up jogging, but found that she had to plan her routes carefully to make sure a restroom would be available along the way. It turned out, after a careful review of her diet and without any specific therapy, that her problem was diet colas. The artificial sweetener had caused a bladder irritation. This is not uncommon nowadays, by the way; but it had eluded all the doctors she had seen.

Or consider something that is happening quite commonly these days in California. After a particularly heavy rainfall, mold tends to form in the heating system of a home. Then, during a cold spell, the forced-air system blasts the bacteria throughout the home. Who is home most of the day to absorb this shower of pollutants? The housewife (homemaker, mother, woman friend, etc.). When a young woman came to me recently with allergylike symptoms, such as a roseate face and sniffles, I tried the whole range of nutrient adjustments with little success. Then she told me she had felt much better on a week's vacation to Mexico. In the old days, the doctor would put this down as a perfect example of psychosomatic illness: take a trip, change your mental outlook. To me, this improvement made me suspect there might be something in the home environment that was causing the symptoms. Sure enough, by changing the filters on the furnace the problem was solved.

Nutritional medicine, you see, is far more than taking large doses of vitamins. It has to do with everything you take into your body: light, noise, air, water, and, of course, food. And there are interactions not only among nutrients, but among the various types of physical stimulants that affect the body. It is now known, for example, that in sexual arousal, certain hormones are released by an interaction of light and zinc. The pineal gland is the mediating link between the eyes and the sex glands; it contains large concentrations of zinc. Studies have shown that sexual intensity may actually be increased by daylight. (It is also well known, by the way, that zinc has other important functions in both male and female sexuality; hence the importance of the food sources of zinc, such as oysters, in fertility and potency.)

In the great majority of patients I treat, nutrient therapy consists primarily of uncovering deficiencies and overcoming them through either food or vitamin/mineral supplements. Nutrient therapy is not a substitute for nor a contradiction of drug therapy. Rather, nutrient therapy is necessarily the first step in dealing with any health problem; drug therapy is the last resort. Nutrients *enable* the biochemistry of the body to work; drugs *block,* in the strict medical sense, one or several elements of that biochemistry. Drugs are often necessary, but no drug should be considered without first exhausting the natural remedies of eliminating poisons and supplying nutrients. Nutrient therapy is the essential foundation for any rational approach to medical care. The fact that in the last two decades of the 20th century most doctors have very little idea of what nutrient therapy is says quite a bit about the sluggishness and obstinacy of the medical bureaucracy. And this is a second major reason why I have chosen to address this book to women.

Women have been the special victims of American medical practice. In *Womancare,* Lynda Madaras and Jane Patterson attribute this to what they call the "M.D.eity" complex of male doctors. Dr. Robert Mendelsohn has been battling the privileged status of physicians in our society for years; in *Male Practice* he takes particular aim at the disasters inflicted on women by a complacent and sexist medical hierarchy. Somewhere between 150,000 and 300,000 hysterectomies performed this year are medically unjustified. Radical mastectomies are only now being questioned on a case-by-case basis. Some 70 percent of the clients of Planned Parenthood take contraceptive pills; less than 9 percent of the female staff of that group do. (The Pill has long been implicated in serious side effects, chiefly heart disease, although recent studies suggest a protective effect in some forms of cancer.) From Dalkon Shields to DES to diuretics for pregnant women, the female of the species has suffered unnecessarily, largely because the male-dominated medico-industrial complex has cared too little about problems uniquely female. Nutrition is an area of medical practice in which women have the opportunity to assert their rights vigorously and effectively.

The advances in nutrient therapy are coming so fast, in all the major health problems of our age, that only a grassroots revolution can bring them to the attention of physicians and into widespread use. Women have the power to organize and successfully carry out such a revolution. Some 70 percent of patients are women. Women dominate the marketplace in choosing and preparing food. As Adelle Davis was the first to discover, women are nutrition-conscious; an A. C. Nielsen survey confirmed a few years ago that a significantly higher percentage of women than men initiate a dietary plan on their own, without the advice of a doctor. Though much publicity has been focused on heart attacks in males, women tend to have the great majority of the most common debilitating diseases: four times the anemia, twice the diabetes, three times the osteoporosis, twice the gallstones, twice the arthritis and three times the rheumatoid arthritis, and *thirty* times the urinary-tract infections. Over the age of forty-five, women tend to be obese more than twice as often as men (among black women, more than *four* times). It's a safe guess that common depression afflicts four times as many women as men, and much more frequently. Women have every reason to look for answers on their own, to not be content to wait for medical advances to trickle down through another generation of medical students. Medical progress is typically 40 years behind the pioneer work.

And the pioneer work in modern medicine is the most exciting and promising in the field of *metabolic* medicine. Consider
these developments, some of which are already taken for
granted among nutrient therapists:

- Chelation therapy with EDTA: Bypass operations can cost
  from $10,000 to $50,000. Many years of clinical experience and recent controlled studies have shown that at less
  than 10 percent of this cost most surgeries of this kind can
  be avoided. The only danger is for patients who have a
  preexisting kidney problem.

- DMSO: This has now become something of a "bootleg
  drug" because of a quite unscientific position of the FDA.
  In spite of four international conferences and more than
  1,200 papers devoted to its safety and efficacy, the regulatory bodies have fallen all over themselves to restrain
  its use. Approved only for a rare bladder disease and a
  few other investigational uses, DMSO has so many
  documented benefits as an anti-inflammatory agent that
  any physician who is not using it is derelict in his or her
  duties.

- Progesterone, a female hormone that is a natural com-
  plement to the other main female hormone, estrogen, has
  now been shown to be effective in a wide variety of wom-
  en's problems, including premenstrual syndrome and infertility. The whole matter of hormones, as we will see in
  Chapter 4, is crucial for women and has been insufficiently
  studied.

- Para amino benzoic acid, or PABA, is an exciting mole-
  cule, a component of folic acid and probably the active
  element in the much-touted "youth" pill Gerivitol, with
  two disparate but important benefits. PABA absorbs ul-
  traviolet light at the right frequency, and so protects the
  skin against the aging effects of overexposure to the sun.
  And, as I have discovered in several interesting cases,
  PABA is also unusually effective against chronic fatigue
  and depression.

Or consider these druglike actions of well-known nutrients.
I would not need to list all these except for the fact that current

medical practice takes little note of them; and even as they are beginning to appear in the "official" journals of orthodox medicine their value is difficult to recognize in the drug-dominated atmosphere of the medical profession.

- Carnitine helps regulate the heartbeat, and thus is helpful in problems of cardiac arrhythmias. It is readily available in good quality meats. As we will see, this amino acid has many promising features.
- Vitamin B_2 (riboflavin) is helpful in preventing and treating cataracts. Its main sources in foods are proteins, especially dairy products.
- Vitamin B_3 (niacin) has recently been shown to protect against diarrhea. Even cholera toxin can be reversed by pre-treatment with niacin, according to recent research at Johns Hopkins Medical Center.
- Vitamin B_6 (pyridoxine) is needed to metabolize protein, and this fact is becoming increasingly important in the face of several conditions in the American diet. Steroid contraceptive pills, for example, so inhibit pyridoxine that diet alone cannot supply it sufficiently. The sterilization needed in some baby formulas has destroyed B_6 to such an extent as to cause convulsions in babies. Old age, drugs, and alcohol place severe demands on this vitamin. The B_6 lost in milling of white flour is *not* replaced by enrichment—and grains are its major dietary source.
- B_{12} has been known for years as a nutrient treatment of asthma. Dr. Jonathan Wright once searched the literature and found several references to this use. Recently a middle-aged woman had to be helped into my office, her asthma attack was so severe; with the use of 1,000 micrograms of B_{12} twice a day she was able to function with only a single use of her inhalant a day. (A microgram is a thousandth of a milligram, which in turn is a thousandth of a gram.) B_{12} is especially important for pregnant women and vegetarians (the latter because the sources of this vitamin are mainly meat and fish). It is false to criticize "megadoses" of vitamins when the effective dose of B_{12} for

asthma is more than 300 times the RDA and when other therapeutic doses of nutrients are equally high.

- Vitamin E was once called the "vitamin in search of a disease." The early researchers in this nutrient now have the last laugh (and they should get Nobel prizes): because it activates the prostaglandins, vitamin E has now been shown in controlled studies to play a key role in protection against atherosclerosis. It is plentiful in oils and nuts, as well as leafy vegetables and unrefined whole wheat.

- Iodine has proved useful in fibrocystic breast disease and as an expectorant; it is available as a supplement in drops, and is found in more normal amounts in seafood.

- Glutathione is an amino acid that is rapidly earning a reputation as a nutrient with the broad application of vitamin C. Recent studies have shown it has more than a dozen known benefits. It can prevent certain cancers, detoxifies heavy metals, deactivates free radicals, ameliorates the harmful effects of radiation, smoking, alcohol, helps against inflammation, and slows the aging process.

I present this imposing list of nutrient effects on the mind and body not to overwhelm you, but to convey some idea of what is going on in mega-nutrition research and clinical practice. In the following chapters I will be going into detail on the nutrients of specific interest to women. As a practicing physician in this field I am impressed by the rapidly changing therapeutics now available for patients. I want to emphasize that in the above list of nutrient therapies (1) all have been confirmed by accepted scientific studies reported in reputable medical journals, and (2) all these advances have occurred within the last few years. And I have not even mentioned those continuing confirmations of the therapeutic effects of such major nutrients as vitamin C and the trace minerals.

The critics of nutrient therapy frequently indulge in a fallacious caricature of the vitamin-conscious person as one who believes that if something is good for you a lot more of it will be even better. This is supposedly a rational critique of megavitamin therapy. There are two facts that this shallow view ignores:

1. The nutrient requirements of *healthy* people can vary from the supposed "normal" level by factors of as much as 30.
2. The nutrient requirements of *sick* people can vary by factors as high as 1,000.

I have mentioned that it takes 300 times the RDA of vitamin B_{12} to be effective against asthma. Dr. Robert Cathcart has shown that doses of 50 or 60 grams of vitamin C—1,000 times the RDA—are needed in some infectious diseases. Folic acid in 10-milligram doses has cured schizophrenia; it would take 10 gallons of orange juice to get that much (and orange juice is a good source). A recent study showed that after surgery approximately 100 times the RDA of vitamin A was needed to prevent the drop in lymphocyte counts. A so-called "toxic" dose of 200 times the RDA of A has proved effective in a severe skin disease—without the expected side effects.

My experience with today's woman patient is that she is not going to accept the useless platitudes of bureaucratic medicine. She is not going to be swayed by vacuous warnings about over-doses of vitamins. I have yet to read of a death attributed to a vitamin overdose; yet three deaths a day are caused by aspirin. I was encouraged by a recent story in *Medical Tribune* about a woman who had enough from American medicine regarding premenstrual syndrome (PMS). "I traveled from Wisconsin to Massachusetts and back again in search of a doctor who would take me seriously," Virginia Cassara said. "Repeatedly, I was told, 'Go home and put another coat of nail polish on, and you'll feel better.'" So she went to London to a clinic founded by Dr. Katharine Dalton, where the treatment is primarily with progesterone. Ms. Cassara has now set up a clearinghouse for women (and doctors) who want more information about the nutritional treatment of PMS.

I suggest that women start organizing around the other major health concerns that affect them as women. And I suggest that more physicians start listening to those concerns. Not all nutrient therapy applies to women alone; and not all women need nutrient therapy. But the odds are heavily in your favor if you look to mega-nutrition as the means to achieving your personal best.

Women are the link between the doctor's office and the supermarket. In an even more obvious way, women are the link between the unborn and the future of society. It is not an easy field—this new combination of nutrition and medicine—to make one's way through. The stakes are enormous. As the authors of *Laurel's Kitchen,* quoted in the epigraph to this book, write:

> The nurturant impulse, the eye for the good of all, may have its most obvious place in a domestic setting, but it is a blessing to hospitals, offices, and classrooms as well. No, I would never go on record as saying, "A woman's place is in the home." But to my mind, the most effective front for social change, the critical point where our efforts will count the most, is not in business or professions, which tackle life's problems from above, from outside, but in the home and community, where the problems start.

These are the larger, social issues mega-nutrition can deal with. Think, for a minute, about the fact that in 1980 we as a nation consumed *four times* the amount of soft drinks, per person, as we did in 1960. That was 38 gallons a year for each of us of sugared water. Go to any college campus and look at what is in every social room or floor landing of a dormitory: a soft-drink machine. Ray Peat tells of seeing miserably poor women in Mexico feeding their babies an American cola drink and a piece of white bread. We are exporters of our nutritional vices.

Somewhere in the mid-70s we passed the point at which half of all the food we eat is *processed.* Of 18,000 items in the average supermarket, some 15,000 are now processed foods. Is it possible for most of us to eat the so-called balanced diet, and get all the nutrients we need, when for most of us the supermarket is our only source of supply? Yes, it is—and we will consider some practical ideas in a later chapter; but it requires considerable diligence. The message of mega-nutrition is *not* to pop a vitamin supplement and then throw anything in your mouth. *Good food selection comes first.* But if you are not clearly in the peak of health—and that means mental alertness, eagerness to work, endurance, full sexuality, and the sense of the joy of living—then a mega-nutritional supplement is probably in order. If you are vaguely ill, but don't know the cause, then a specific vitamin-mineral deficiency analysis is in order. If you have a serious medical problem, you must see a doctor; but you and your doctor must also restore your nutritional status before anyone intervenes with drugs or surgery.

The malnutrition factor (and we now know that half the people in this country are deficient in some known nutrient) is compounded by the pollution factor. This malnutrition/ pollution factor is the premise of mega-nutrition's prescription for a good vitamin/mineral supplement each day. Adelle Davis once wrote that such supplements are too expensive and that food is the first choice. She's right about the latter, but nowadays a supplement is very good insurance at a relatively reasonable cost.

There is one further motivation in this cause that must appeal especially to the nurturant impulses of women. It has been expressed best by the late René Dubos:

> It seems reasonable to envisage a time when dietary regimens can be designed not only for growth and health, but for certain physiological functions and cultural values. When, and if, we can reach the proper level of knowledge, nutrition will become part of a new science—as yet undeveloped—of human ecology.

2

Listen to Your Body
—Your Personal Diet
—Your Crisis Diet

This is the first new diet in more than a century! I can make this claim after seeing patient after patient go through one highly publicized diet after another with little lasting success. If any one of these diets had any basic merit, it would have lasted longer than a fad. The Listen to Your Body diet is easy to follow without any special formulas, without long charts of favored foods, without special recipes. All other diets make the simple mistake of trying to dish up the same program to everyone. Only the Listen to Your Body diet is personal, because only this diet relies on a basic adjustment of the three food types, for you alone! And only this approach gives you a *crisis* diet with complete safety. (See page 38.)

It's this easy: First you're going to learn about carbohydrates. You're going to eliminate carbohydrates completely from your diet, then bring them back in a controlled way until you reach the ideal level *for you*. Second, you're going to learn how to adjust your fats and proteins. Third, you're going to learn to *listen* for the key signals that tell you when you have reached your personal best level of all three food types.

The reason why this diet will last, will not become just another fad, is that it teaches you the most important things about nutrition as you go along. Because it is so basic, it provides the four basic things a diet should:

1. Quick, safe weight loss
2. Weight control
3. Mood improvement
4. Beauty enhancement

To begin, follow the text and look at the diagrams.

PHASE ONE
The Personal Carbohydrate Adjustment
Test for Your Personal Best!

1. For two days eat only foods from the Non-carbohydrate List below. This establishes a condition known as *ketosis.** Ketones are the by-products of the breakdown of fats—when the body runs out of carbohydrates. Ketones are used by the body for fuel—for the brain, heart, and muscles—when other food sources are gone (such as in starvation). So they are not just a waste product. The only precaution you need to take during these two days is to make sure you have ample potassium—and this is easily done by using Morton's Lite Salt on your food. Diabetics should exercise caution, since they are generally unable to handle carbohydrates properly to begin with. There are minor amounts of carbohydrate in this list, but after two days you essentially will be at "ground zero" as far as your carbohydrate intake is concerned.

- NON-CARBOHYDRATE LIST
  You may eat all types of meat, fish, fowl, cheese, eggs, and fats, including butter and oil. You should also eat a total of as much as two cups a day of salad and salad vegetables: Lettuce, cabbage, parsley, watercress, celery, cucumber, asparagus, broccoli, zucchini, eggplant, olives, and avocado *bits*. You *must* drink liquids—six or more glasses a day of *only*: water, mineral water, club soda, or tea. Notice what this *excludes*: No alcohol, coffee, seasonings such as sugar, honey, catsup, lemon juice; no vegetables other than the ones listed; no grains of any kind. There are no limits, however, to the quantities of foods from the above list.

2. On the third day begin adding carbohydrate foods in a controlled way. Add 6 grams per meal, or 18 grams per day, using the Graded Carbohydrate List on the following page.

---

* There is a simple method of determining if you are in ketosis, which may appeal to women who want to be exact. You can purchase a small box of Ketostix at any pharmacy and follow the directions to measure the appearance of ketones. For most people, however, the two-day rule is quite sufficient. Do not be misled by any vague warnings about the dangers of ketosis, such as bad breath. For some people, a breath *change* occurs, which in severe cases can be overcome with a mouthwash.

- GRADED CARBOHYDRATE LIST (Add 18 grams per day)
    3-gram foods: ½ large tomato, 4 lettuce leaves, ¼ avocado, ½ cup mushrooms or sprouts, 1 Tbsp peanut butter
    6-gram foods: 1 oz (20) nuts, ¼ cantaloupe, ½ cup berries, ½ cup carrots, 1 cup coleslaw, green beans, soy curd, or cottage cheese, 6 oz tomato juice, 1 Tbsp wheat germ or brewer's yeast, 2 Tbsp bran, 1 tsp sugar or honey*
    12-gram foods: 1 cup milk, 1 slice bread, 1 apple or orange, ½ grapefruit, 12 grapes, ½ cup nuts, 1 cup plain yogurt
    24-gram foods: 1 medium potato, ½ cup peas, beans, grains, rice, or noodles, 1 large banana, 1 cup orange juice, ½ cup fruit yogurt, a 1-oz candy bar, 1 slice cake, 1 scoop ice cream, 3 prunes or ¼ cup raisins, 1 small pear, an 8-oz cola drink

3. On each day write down the foods eaten and how you feel.

Remember, keep it simple! Don't worry about exact weights or small variations among foods—such as the difference between almonds and cashews. After seven days (five on increasing carbohydrates) you will be at a level of 90–100 grams of carbohydrate a day. Keep increasing carbohydrates from the above list until you feel you have passed the point at which you "feel best." Use the nine Listen Factors listed in Phase Three to help decide which day is your best. Now remain at this level of carbohydrate intake as you enter the second phase.

PHASE TWO
The Personal Fat and Protein Adjustment

1. Make sure of adequate protein. You need approximately 1 gram of protein for every 2 pounds of your *ideal* weight. So if you want to weigh 137 pounds, your body needs about 68

---

* Note that sugar, honey and processed foods are generally considered "simple carbohydrates." Fruits and vegetables are "complex." Complex carbohydrates are better sources of nutrients and fiber. (See page 33.)

grams of protein per day. To make sure you are getting adequate protein, use the Protein Equivalency List below.

● PROTEIN EQUIVALENCY LIST

7 grams: 1 egg, 1 cup milk, 1 oz cheese, ½ cup beans, 1 cup cooked wheat or rice
14 grams: 3 oz high-fat meat, ½ cup cottage cheese
21 grams: 3 oz fish or low-fat meat

2. Adjust for fats, up or down, by choosing your carbohydrate foods (mainly vegetables) and your non-carbohydrate foods (mainly animal) from the Animal-Vegetable Fat List below.

● ANIMAL-VEGETABLE FAT LIST

ANIMAL

HIGH FAT	LOW–MEDIUM FAT
Beef, lamb, pork: 3 oz (24)*	Fish, skinned fowl, veal, liver, brains: 3 oz (8)
Lard, butter: 1 Tbsp (16)	Sweetbreads: 3 oz (4)
2 eggs, 2 cups milk, 2 oz cheese: (16)	Low-fat milk or yogurt, low-fat cottage or ricotta cheese: 8 oz (virtually 0)
Fowl, with skin: 3 oz (16)	

VEGETABLE

HIGH FAT	LOW–MEDIUM FAT
Nuts, seeds: 2 Tbsp (8)	Grains: ½ cup (2)
½ avocado, 4 olives: (8)	Beans: ½ cup (1)
Vegetable oils, margarine: 1 Tbsp (16)	Bread: 1 slice (1)
	Leaves, yeast, green beans, stems, roots, tubers, broccoli, peas, melon, squash, berries, vegetable juice, fruit juice: 1 cup (virtually 0)

* Numbers in parentheses refer to grams of fat. To estimate caloric intake, assume that a pound of fat has about twice as many calories as a pound of either protein or carbohydrate.

PHASE THREE
Learning to Listen

Adjust your fats and carbohydrates in response to the messages from your body. Use the Listen Factor List below.

● LISTEN FACTOR LIST

Hunger Increase fats from high-fat vegetable list, or decrease carbohydrate intake.

Craving sweets Increase carbohydrate a little, up to 30 grams extra per day.

Weakness Increase potassium: use Morton's Lite Salt or natural sources such as berries, squash, melon, or vegetable juice.

Headache Increase potassium as above, or lower carbohydrates.

Lightheadedness Increase potassium as above, or add protein.

Irritability Increase carbohydrate 30 grams; if irritability persists, try a low level again (10–40 grams a day).

Fatigue Increase protein from low-fat animal list.

Constipation Increase potassium as above, or add vegetable fiber.

No weight loss Eat proteins first. Increase exercise to burn calories and metabolize fats better. Reduce calories by choosing from low-fat lists. Choose high-fiber vegetables from the low-fat list. To achieve weight gain, reverse any or all of these.

Note that I have simplified the portions and values of common carbohydrate, protein, and fat foods so that the gram-amounts are respectively in multiples of 6, 7, and 8. This will aid in remembering basic values. Again, I stress that you keep it *simple*. A kitchen scale is not necessary. If you are faced with onerous details, you may miss the basic idea of the program.

PHASE ONE
Carbohydrate Adjustment

	1st Day	**2nd Day**
EMPTY YOUR-SELF OF CARBO-HYDRATES.	Eat any meat, fish, dairy item, butter, oil. Salads up to 2 cups (incl. asparagus, olives, broccoli, zucchini, etc.) Drink 6 glasses water, club soda, tea *only*	Same as 1st Day. Remember: *no* alcohol, sugar, catsup, bread, or other vegetables. You should reach ketosis—showing fats are being burned

	3rd Day	**4th Day**
ADD CARBO-HYDRATES BACK A LITTLE AT A TIME. TAKE NOTES ON HOW YOU FEEL (SEE LIST).	Add 6 g carbo-hydrates each meal. Example: ¼ melon at breakfast, 1 cup cottage cheese at lunch, ¼ avocado and ½ large tomato at dinner	Add 6 g carbo-hydrates *more* each meal. Example: 1 cup milk (12), 1 slice bread (12), ½ cup raisins (12), 6 oz tomato juice (6) with ½ cup green beans
	You are at 18 g per day	*You are at 36 g per day*

5th Day	**6th Day**	**7th Day**
Add 6 g carbo-hydrates *more* each meal. Example: ½ cup berries (6) with 1 tbsp wheat germ (6) and 1 tsp. honey (6), 1 apple (12) with 1 cup coleslaw (6). 2 tbsp bran (6) with 1 cup yogurt (12)	Add 6 g carbo-hydrates *more* each meal. Example: 1 medium potato (24) 1 large banana (24) ½ cup peas, beans (24) ½ cup *fruit* yogurt (24) ¼ cup raisins (24) 1 scoop ice cream (24)	Add 6 g carbo-hydrates *more* each meal. Example: 2 tbsp peanut butter (6), 2 tsp jelly (12), 1 slice bread (12), or 1 slice cake (24) with 6 grapes (6), or 1 cup orange juice (24) with 1 tbsp brewer's yeast (6)
You are at 54 g per day	*You are at 72 g per day*	*You are at 90 g per day*

PHASE TWO
Fat and Protein Adjustment

	8th day	**9th day**
FIX PERSONAL CARBO-HYDRATE LEVEL. CHECK PROTEIN (SEE LIST). INDULGE IN FATS.	Go back to the carbohydrate level at which you felt best (18, 36, 54, 72, 90, or add more). Add up your protein to make sure you have ½ your weight (lbs.) in protein (gms)	Keep carbohydrates steady. Now choose *high* fat protein and carbohydrates. E.g.: meat, nuts, avocado, oils

You are now at ____ carbohydrates   *You are still at ____ carbohydrates*

10th day

CUT DOWN FATS. KEEP CARBOHY-DRATES CONSTANT	Continue to keep carbohydrates same. Now choose *low* fat protein and carbohydrates. E.g.: dairy items, fish, skinned fowl, organ meats. very low: cottage cheese, skim milk, grains, most vegetables and fruit

You are still at ____ carbohydrates

Write down: Your personal best carbohydrate level ____ (8th day)
              Your personal best fat level ____ (9th or 10th day)

PHASE THREE
Listen to Your Body

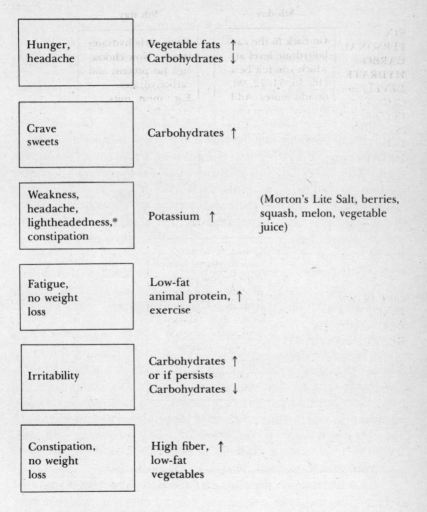

Hunger, headache	Vegetable fats ↑ Carbohydrates ↓	
Crave sweets	Carbohydrates ↑	
Weakness, headache, lightheadedness,* constipation	Potassium ↑	(Morton's Lite Salt, berries, squash, melon, vegetable juice)
Fatigue, no weight loss	Low-fat animal protein, ↑ exercise	
Irritability	Carbohydrates ↑ or if persists Carbohydrates ↓	
Constipation, no weight loss	High fiber, ↑ low-fat vegetables	

* Try extra protein as well

When Should You Go on a Diet?

You see how logical and easy my dietary program is. Now you must ask yourself, Is it for me? Am I overweight? Am I interested primarily in feeling better? Am I willing to take action *on my own behalf*? These questions may seem on the surface to call for an immediate and resounding YES, but, of course, little is that simple in "real" life, especially for women.

Women are caught right in the middle of the diet struggle. On one hand they are cajoled by societal pressures and advertising to conform to the "right" weight and shape; on the other hand they have special nutritional responsibilities, usually to their families but at least to themselves, by virtue of being female. Thus it is not uncommon to see teenagers and young women depleted in minerals such as iron as they attempt to limit their calories to 1,200 a day in a weight-reduction program. And it is not uncommon to hear mothers asking about the dangers of butter and eggs and whole milk as they daily face the barrage of simplistic cholesterol-scare advertising. Women seem to be tiptoeing gingerly through a minefield of forbidden foods in our society. As Oscar Wilde said, tongue in cheek, "Women have more fun in life than men: more things are forbidden them."

Have such pressures always existed, or are women only now set on a sort of collision course of good nutrition and thinness? There are probably cycles in this as there are in fashion. But it is also likely that we are seeing something more dangerous for women in our current preoccupation with diet—paradoxically because we are learning more and more about nutrition. There are now more things to be afraid of, or at least so we are told. And there are major clashes in nutritional philosophy these days: are fats the villain, or is it carbohydrates?

"The tyranny of slenderness," as Kim Chernin terms our current diet malaise, may be in for a rebellion. Ms. Chernin describes her arrival at the University of California in the early 1960s as chained to her tape measure, calorie counter, and scales. But now she finds women reacting as she does to dieting. "It's unnatural and unhealthy. . . . We call it controlling hunger, but what is that hunger? What some women are really trying to control is an assertiveness that they've been taught is dangerous." The feminist aspect of this view of dieting is quite explicit. Again, Ms. Chernin: "This whole question of the body's reduction is analogous to the binding of women's feet in prerevolutionary China." The models in *Vogue* may have sunken cheeks and prepubescent bodies for years to come, but the change that Ms. Chernin senses has already been reflected in a revision in the "ideal" weight charts used by insurance companies. The ideal is now several pounds heavier, for height and body type, than it has been all these years.

What I am leading up to is not some "eat what you like" diet, or "fat is beautiful," but to a dietary approach that can lead women out of the unnecessary dilemma between good looks and good nutrition. Stating the problem is tantamount to solving it: good looks *come from,* and are not opposed to, good nutrition. Why this is so, and how you can put this truth to work for you for a lifetime, are the subjects of the rest of this chapter.

Men Are More Like Women than Women Are Like Women

This maxim that every woman is surprisingly different from the woman next door, is basic to the plan that is the culmination of all my dietary work in nutrition. As a psychiatrist as well as a nutritionist and general practitioner, I have looked at both sides of the problem of weight loss (and sometimes weight gain). I can appreciate what women like Kim Chernin have to say about the unconscious pressures that men put on women in our society. I also know how psychological and physical problems tend to overlap or merge with such basic human needs as the desire to be attractive and the wish for good health. Most importantly, as one of the founders and as the past president of the Orthomolecular Medical Society (OMS), I have had to organize seminars, publish bulletins, and generally chart a course for "the new medicine" within the framework of existing medical practice. In this connection I've organized and refereed debates between the leading exponents of low-fat and low-carbohydrate diets. I've had to sift through thousands of medical periodicals for clues to the honest truth about everything the OMS does; for when anyone proposes a therapy that goes beyond conventional practice he or she had better be right. I may not have all the answers, but I have been in a unique position to review and evaluate what is known on the subject of *diet*.

From all this experience I've set up a dietary program for my patients that has now been checked out for more than ten years. It is this practical experience, backed by research now being done in the field of bariatrics (the study of weight control) that is the basis for the Listen to Your Body diet. It works. It's not a craze or a gimmick. It's the answer to psychological as well as physical health problems, including weight loss. And it's especially meant for *women*.

Why especially for women? First, any diet plan that does not take good health into account misses the basic problem I have described as the dilemma between good looks and good nutrition. Men don't face that dilemma, for the most part. Second, as the maxim in the above heading is meant to convey, there is a far greater diversity among women than among men. In the first chapter I stressed the importance of biochemical individuality. The range of nutritional, which is to say *biochemical*, needs in women is quite a bit wider than such a range in men. (One obvious example—some women are mothers of large families, some never bear children.) Even a casual glance at a text on gynecology is enough to show the vast differences from one woman's health concerns to the next one's. The Listen to Your Body diet is the only dietary plan that takes this diversity into proper account.

Learning About Eating the Easy Way

All the diet books I've seen have one feature in common: nutrition is a sort of necessary evil in the discussion. You are supposed to be awed by the scientific references, then forget them as you plunge ahead with the recipes. The Listen to Your Body diet is quite different in this respect: it's a way of teaching you about foods and good eating habits. Once you have gone through the three stages of this diet you will know more about nutrition than most nutritionists, and you will never have to refer to a table again—except your *dinner* table.

It is not surprising that Jean Mayer, formerly of Harvard,

now president of Tufts and a well-known syndicated columnist, had this to say of the state of nutrition education:

> Our studies at Harvard suggest that the average physician knows a little more about nutrition than the average secretary—unless the secretary has a weight problem. Then she probably knows more than the average physician.

The nutritional value of foods can be listed in charts or tables, broken down by food type, in some comparable portions. You may discover, and remember, that parsley is an excellent source of Vitamin C; but to eat a cup of parsley? Even a full cup of an ordinary vegetable, such as green beans, is quite a portion. Yet the Food and Drug Administration allows canners of green beans to give RDA values for green beans in terms of 1-cup portions. Or one can look up the major vitamins and minerals in a reference book and see what foods are their major sources. You might find, for example, that a cup of raisins provides 0.35 milligrams of vitamin B_6 (not a bad source—better than brown rice, broccoli, or wheat germ); but then you notice that the RDA for an adult is 2 milligrams—*six times* as much. If you selected one of the better sources of B_6, kale, you would have to eat a pound and a half of it (raw) to get your RDA.

A third way of learning something about nutrition is to consult the occasional "super foods" lists. I feel that such a rating system, like a one-to-four star system in restaurant reviews, can be helpful. But is there much to be learned when such a list fails to take *you* into account? For example, a list I recently saw in a consumer's co-op ranked vegetables by the *number* of RDAs each one supplied in significant amounts. A vegetable that gives you 25 percent of the RDA for Vitamin A, 30 percent for C, and 40 percent for thiamine is a "3." On this basis, collard greens and corn-on-the-cob were ranked as "super veggies." Black-eyed peas, kale, turnip greens, parsley, and spinach were runners-up. Mustard greens, okra, red peppers, lima beans, broccoli, peas, and asparagus came next. Even if you remembered these distinctions, what would this tell you about any one nutrient you might particularly need? And if you or your children simply don't like the stuff, how much would get off the plate and into the appropriate mouth?

So I'm really making two pleas here: first, a diet plan must be practical, must take your eating habits and likes and dislikes into account; second, such a plan must be specific, must take your *particular* physical and emotional needs into account. Add to this the third variable—what I have called the "biological complexity of food"—and you have indeed an imposing problem. What's the answer?

Traditionally, doctors have preached *variety* in eating habits as the only practical solution. In effect they've said, "We just can't know our particular needs accurately enough, and we just can't remember, even if we knew, the biochemical contribution of foods. So if we range over the whole spectrum of fruits, vegetables, and animal sources of food, we're likely to pick up all the micronutrients we need, regardless of our vast individual differences." This method is, in fact, what our appetites tell us to do; we naturally tend to like variety. Even if we all had a lobster budget, few of us would choose lobster more than a few times a week. So it would seem that we *can* let nature take its course. Is this what the Listen diet comes down to?

Not at all. Again, there is a practical problem—we do not live in an ideal world, or anything close to it. Several factors in our current evolution as human beings, as well as several man-made contributions to our environment, *interfere with* the signals our bodies send to us. In some obvious cases, our cravings are overpowering, and we can assume such hungers are so biologically urgent that even the static of environmental pollution and overprocessing of food can't disguise the message. Pregnant women, for example, have a variety of unusual cravings in the course of their pregnancies. Why pickles? I once suggested in an offhand way that perhaps the pregnant woman really wants the trace minerals in the brine solution, and not the pickles at all. The more I analyze the tremendous demands that the fetus places on the expectant mother, the more I have come to appreciate the power of the "biological telegraph system" in a woman's body.

This may seem obvious to any woman, yet, unbelievably, only a few years ago gynecologists were giving diuretics to pregnant women in a misguided effort to hold down their weight. These medications were literally washing mineral salts away from the developing fetus. This is a scandal that has received far too little publicity, but the effects of such mineral depletion on the fetus are merely *less obvious, not less serious*, than the horrors of thalidamide or diethylstilbestrol (DES). How quickly we assimilate the new knowledge of the dangerous effects of drugs, and forget how "science" was telling us there was nothing to be concerned about! Dr. Ben Siegel of the University of Oregon Medical School recalled recently that only 25 years ago X-rays were routinely taken of pregnant women without a thought about possible dangers to the unborn. He was then working at the Virus Laboratory at the University of California at Berkeley and attended a conference at which Linus Pauling suggested that X-rays might cause genetic damage to the fetus. The doctors in the room and the scientific community outside it scoffed at such a bizarre idea. Just another wild speculation by Dr. Pauling!

How Poor Foods Drive Out Good Foods

Food processing also masks the signals we should be getting from food and from our bodies with typically heavy use of salt and sugar. Even our baby foods were once thoroughly salted and sugared, and as we grew we became used to foods like catsup that contained (and still contain) large amounts of sweeteners, as well as to soups, mayonnaise, peanut butter, and even canned and frozen vegetables liberally "filled" with sucrose. We didn't worry about canned fruits floating in heavy syrup, and only recently have consumers risen up against breakfast "foods" that contain more sugar than candy bars. Over the years we have grown so used to salt on nuts, snacks, and all sorts of canned goods that when we sample an unsalted version we think something is wrong. Now there are good reasons why the food industry has relied on salt and sugar in processing: both are excellent preservatives (sugar is so devoid of nutrients that not even microbes can live in it). Sugar is also one of the cheapest "fillers," volume for volume, that a manufacturer can use to extend his product. Once started down this path, processors discovered that the basic sweet and salt flavors had an almost addictive effect on consumers—hence the ludicrous extremes of ready-to-eat children's cereals. Needing nutrients to be digested, an "empty calorie" food like sugar can be dangerous; and, although salt in itself in moderation is not dangerous to most people, we do know that when potassium levels in the body are low, sodium can in fact cause widespread problems. In addition to all this, my concern with salt and sugar here is that they both hinder our ability to *listen*. Quite simply, they pervert our taste buds.

It goes without saying that smoking dulls our sensitivity to tastes. But so do a lot of pollutants beyond our control: smog, pesticides, industrial wastes. To prepare ourselves to hear what our cravings are telling us, we may have to get rid of some bad habits and make sure that we are getting enough of the micronutrients that protect against pollutants.

Many of us, in addition, have allergies that can mask our food cravings. Finally, most of us confuse our appetite controls by not getting sufficient exercise. As Dr. Tom Bassler says, "Sedentary people have very dumb stomachs." When we leave unburned calories in our bodies from the previous day, looking for storage places, our stomachs fail to give us definite signals on what to eat. So we eat blindly. It is Bassler's observation that marathon runners crave whole grains and vegetables, nuts, onions, garlic, and fresh fruits—more so than non-runners—because their appetites are not dulled by the hormonal mechanisms of storing food. Satiety dulls us; hunger sharpens our senses. Thus, long-distance runners are known to start burning fat as well as carbohydrates after an hour or so of exercise; hence a noticeable craving for fatty, even greasy foods after extended runs. As we will see in Chapter 10, exercise has a greater role to play than the simple burning of calories (strictly speaking, we should say "burning of *nutrients*"—of which the unit of measure is calories).

The study of food cravings is a new science (not yet well researched in medical literature), but these brief outlines of how food cravings are masked give you an idea of the enormous importance of what is to be learned. What we have seen is that there are four preliminaries to the Listen to Your Body diet:

1. Concentrate on unprocessed foods so you can be sure the foods you crave contain the nutrients that cause the craving.

2. Reduce your sugar and salt intake, both directly and by cutting down on processed foods, to keep your taste buds intact.
3. Deal with pollutants both by avoiding them wherever possible and by insuring a daily intake of protective micronutrients.
4. Take corrective action against allergies and against a sedentary lifestyle to give your body a chance to "talk" to you.

With this lengthy preamble, we're now ready to look at the "fine tuning" that you can make to adapt the Listen to Your Body diet to your specific needs.

The Dietary Secret Is to Adjust, Not to Avoid or Reduce Fats and Carbohydrates

I have no quarrel with people who like to create diets. Every magazine has one of its own, at least once a year. Movie stars have them. Cities have them. Police departments and air forces and even doctors have them. Most of them are based on menus and recipes rather than on theory, but you can also be sure that no bariatric discovery of the slightest importance will go unpublished by some diet creator. Thus we have seen the fructose diet, based on the interesting fact that this sweetener has less propensity to trigger the cycle of blood sugar ups and downs associated with sucrose. And other diets claim to be based on means of increasing the body's ability to burn fat. Some diet devisers dream up "scientific discoveries" to buttress their regimens, such as Judy Mazel's recently popular Beverly Hills diet. I have no quarrel even with these bizarre creations, because strangely enough they *do* work—simply because they either cause people to stop and think about their food, or they get people off an even worse program.

What I have a great quarrel with is any diet that categorically forbids a major *type* of food. Even the medical establishment is guilty of this, with the "heart diet," as we shall see. Another egregious example is the all-protein diet, usually in liquid form, that has actually killed people.

Consider what happened in the case of the three most popular diets in recent years. Judy Mazel was roundly criticized by the experts for being utterly unscientific. The reaction of Dr. Philip L. White, of the AMA's Department of Foods and Nutrition, was typical: "Her nutrition theory is out of the 19th century, and the diet is dangerous because it's so low in important nutrients and protein." The nutrition department of the University of California Medical School protested the serialization of Miss Mazel's book in the *San Francisco Chronicle* for the same reason, declaring that all calories are the same and that weight reduction is possible only by lowering caloric intake below caloric expenditure. As we will see, her critics were not much more scientific than she was.

Then the long-smoldering feud between Nathan Pritikin and Dr. Robert Atkins came to the surface in a debate on national television. Pritikin claimed that Atkin's low-carbohydrate plan inevitably means high animal fat and the consequent risk of heart disease. Atkins claimed success in treating a wide variety of illnesses with his high-nutrient program, and called the severe Pritikin diet impractical for most people. Dr. White threw up his hands at them both, saying, "I've never 'won' a TV debate with a diet author. They're entertainers. Next to them, we scientific types seem boring—or opposed to new ideas."

Pritikin's Longevity Institute has a remarkable record of success, but primarily with known heart patients. The complete or near-complete restriction of fat in his program is a drastic measure, and only those threatened with a serious ailment can ordinarily motivate themselves to stick to it. Moreover, who is to say what is the basic reason for the success of those who *do* stick to the plan—is it the absence of fat, or the abundance of nutrients that necessarily come with a complex carbohydrate diet? I suggested the latter possibility to Mr. Pritikin during his debate with Dr. Atkins at a convention of the Orthomolecular Medical Society several years ago. Since then, I have also come to suspect that long-term deprivation of nutrients available only or mainly in fats—essential fatty acids (EFAs)—could have serious effects in other physiological problems. Dr. Bassler, who has worked with several patients at the Pritikin center, recently reported to the *New England Journal of Medicine* that the deaths of certain runners might be attributable to "nutritional arrhythmias," or malfunctioning of the electrical timing of the heart muscle—due to chronic depletion of fats. At this stage I am prepared to say that, except for a small percentage of the population suffering from a unique inability to properly utilize fats, a program of drastic fat reduction as proposed by Nathan Pritikin appears misguided.

The Atkins diet has also been characterized in extreme terms, but, I think, unfairly. While calling for a restriction in carbohydrates, he has not recommended a binge on animal fats. My main point is that no one diet is right for everyone, and therefore no doctor or biochemist or exercise therapist can categorically recommend a reduction in any major type of food for the public at large.

What I recommend is just this: First, a carbohydrate adjustment; next, a fat adjustment, keeping protein up and carbohydrates stable, and paying careful attention all along to your energy and your mood.

How you make these adjustments is easy, though perhaps not as easy as the all-this or all-that diets so common in popular magazines. But the effort is worth it, because when you are done you will have not only a tailor-made diet but also a very practical course in nutrition! You will know what you need to know about food.

Ironically, if you cut out fat entirely you may miss an essential oil, linoleic acid, which helps burn fat more quickly! Another helpful fact: in a weight-loss program it's better to eat protein first in the day and even in a meal. Why? Because protein is essential and sweets are not. Both fat and protein turn off hunger, while carbohydrate turns it on.

These are some of the things you may not see at first glance in the protein-fat-carbohydrate lists at the beginning of this chapter:

- The low-fat carbohydrates such as grains, beans, roots, and stems are filling and satisfying, and they also generally contain good quality fiber. (Leaves are also complex carbohydrates, but not as high in fiber.) In choosing carbohydrates rely on them rather than on the fruits (fruit sugars whet the appetite).

- Virtually every grain or vegetable has some protein; fruits have practically none.
- Animal foods provide protein more readily than non-animal foods.
- To lower fats, choose your protein from lean meat, fish, and the legumes.
- Remember that the legumes are quite high in carbohydrates—you'll have to watch them carefully at the first stage of the program.
- For weight reduction it is better to eat snacks rather than meals. A snack is defined as any one or two items in the lists. A "meal" is three different items served together. Anything beyond that is a "feast." Studies have shown that "meals" or "feasts" contribute to more storage of fat than "snacks" of the same caloric value. Five or six "mini-meals" are better than three regular meals with the same total calories.

Protein Deficiency: Not a False Alarm

The issue of protein usually comes up in a discussion of vegetarianism. I read recently in a book about elephants that these prodigious animals must eat 16 hours a day to get enough nourishment—because they are vegetarians. Now there are many admirable things about vegetarians, from a philosophical as well as nutritional point of view. Moreover, in this country those who make this dietary choice do so with their eyes wide open and with a true dedication to good nutritional practices. Yet there are dangers in going overboard on anything—including criticism of meat-eaters.

Protein deficiency is not at all uncommon in the sense that it occurs as frequently as many of the other ailments that bring people to physicians. Yet popular writers on the subject continue to barrage us with stories about athletes who are vegetarians, and with the claim that "a normal diet usually contains excess protein." One book goes so far as to state, "The average of 90 to 100 grams of protein that each person in this country eats each day is almost double what he or she needs." The generally recognized medical rule, however, is that an adult needs about one gram of protein for each two pounds of body weight. (See page 18.) Children need proportionately more for proper growth.

It's the usual vegetarian claim that 40 to 60 grams a day of protein is sufficient. Even if the population of the United States averages 90 to 100 grams, does this mean that we're all getting enough? (People drown in rivers with an *average* depth of two feet, you know.)

Vegetarians agree that one must watch protein intake especially carefully if dairy products as well as red meat, chicken, and fish are excluded from the diet. Random food selection can be highly dangerous over an extended period of time. In a 100-gram serving (about 3½ ounces), there should be at least 2 grams of protein for a food to make a significant contribution to daily protein intake. The following vegetables fail this test: beets, cabbage, carrots, cassava, eggplant, endive, lettuce, pumpkin, sweet potatoes, tomatoes, and turnips. In other ways, these vegetables may appear highly desirable to a dieter. Each is a good source of one or more vitamins and trace minerals, as well as fiber. In trying to get enough fiber, one can easily concentrate on such things as grains, roots, and stems, and so miss out on adequate protein.

Are Some Calories Better than Others?

The weight-loss strategy involved in the Listen diet is quite a bit more than simple caloric reduction. Yes, some calories are better than others—that is, the foods represented by those numbers are burned differently in the body. After all, the metabolism of food is not quite the same as the burning of a woodpile. Biologist Raymond Peat writes, "The fact is that for many people 100 calories of sugar is profoundly different from 100 calories of protein, even when both are taken as excess food beyond an adequate diet. The sugar will affect not only the way it is used, but it will modify the body so that the other food is not used properly." When the empty calories of refined white flour and sugar overstimulate the pancreas, energy is expended in nonproductive ways. The body deposits fat instead of burning it in normal bodily activities. Dr. Peat also points out that an active brain can burn about half of all the energy consumed by the body. Thus, when excessive carbohydrates depress brain activity, food will be stored as fat just as surely as when there is no physical activity to compensate for excessive intake of calories. Proteins and certain fatty acids also vary considerably from one to the next in their ability to "burn" in the body. This characteristic is called their "specific dynamic action."

Why then do all the debunkers of diets—they tend mainly to be establishment spokesmen—insist that "a calorie is a calorie," and that unless one lowers caloric intake or increases physical exercise no weight loss can occur? Well, in a certain sense they are right. One must burn calories to shed pounds (about 4,000 calories per pound). But there are at least four different reasons why some nutrients, in some bodies, burn better than others *without overt physical activity*. And these four ways add up to substantial differences in our ability to lose weight. They are not gimmicks dreamed up by promoters of special pills or special diets; they have all been reported in the leading medical literature for some time.

I have referred briefly to two of these four factors already: (1) the specific dynamic action of certain proteins, and (2) the superiority of foods which do not overstimulate the pancreas (among other internal organs). A third factor in weight gain not explainable by caloric intake is simply a depressed metabolic rate. Studies published in *Nature* in 1979 and in the *New England Journal of Medicine* in 1980 indicate that the obese gain weight at a relatively low daily caloric intake because they have a greater efficiency for storing food energy. The implication is that all of us have a certain regulator that decides when we will burn and when we will store fat. Further studies have suggested that this regulatory mechanism is affected by diet as well as by heredity or illness. Several researchers have confirmed that one's "set point" can be lowered or raised by the quality of food we eat and by exercise habits.

Finally, the fourth factor that influences caloric expenditure without overt corresponding physical activity is . . . exercise. This must seem like a contradiction, but read on! You've seen the tables that tell how many calories are burned in walking, jogging, playing handball, etc. That's the overt physical activity. In addition to that expenditure, *certain types* of exercise cause an ongoing caloric expenditure. A study in the *American Journal of Clinical Nutrition* as far back as 1967 showed that exercise performed for more than an hour nearly doubles the basic metabolic rate (BMR). It runs the motor, so to speak, without the motor's being plugged in—so the motor must be running off its internal batteries. Furthermore, studies in *Lancet* in 1972 and in 1978 showed that aerobic exercise (such as long-distance walking, running, swimming, cycling) establishes certain metabolic pathways for the burning of fat. And *these pathways remain open long after the exercise is completed.* A marathoner can loll about in the comforting knowledge that she's burning more fat than her tennis-playing friends.

Finally, let me elaborate on the Listen Factors; they will be easier to experience if your level of physical activity is high:

Craving sweets This occurs most commonly at the low end of your carbohydrate-reduction program. Your blood sugar may be too low. But hold off on the candy; instead, increase carbohydrates from the Graded Carbohydrate List (page 18) gradually. Try to keep the increase to a maximum of 30 extra grams a day, because that should do it.

General hunger The first reaction is to resume the old eating habits, but we can be quite a bit more specific. First, try a little increase in the fats from the high-fat vegetable list; you'll remember that fats have a tendency to fill the stomach longer. Then *decrease* your carbohydrates. You may still have the wrong mood level, or the carbohydrates may be blocking the hunger-satisfying effect of the fats.

Fatigue More protein is needed, without additional fat. So look in the low-fat animal list—cottage cheese or fish and low-fat meats.

Weakness This feeling is quite different from fatigue. It is the sensation of lack of strength rather than lack of endurance. The sodium-potassium balance may be upside-down, so look for more potassium from the low-fat vegetables—such as berries, squash, or vegetable juice. Or switch to a salt substitute, such as Morton's Lite Salt. Lightheadedness is a feeling that shouldn't be confused with dizziness, which can result from numerous illnesses. Added protein can be helpful for that lightheaded feeling, in addition to the above.

Headache Again, increase potassium, but from the low-carbohydrate list if possible (avocado, meat, etc.). In other cases, simply lowering carbohydrates is effective.

The Listen to Your Body Crisis Diet

These are some of the crises that have brought women to me for something faster, more drastic, or more specific than my "personal diet":

- *Confusion.* Are you unable to deal with the carbohydrate-fat-protein discussion in my basic diet? Many women as well as men find it one chore too much. They want something simple in their complex lives.
- *Time.* Is your life so busy that you can't take time for normal meal preparation—without resorting to junk foods? Many working women with children find this to be so.
- *Results.* Do you want action *fast*? Do you have a timetable that requires quick weight loss in a matter of days rather than weeks or months? There are many good reasons for wanting to see results quickly.
- *Morale.* Have you failed to keep to a diet in the past because of mixed results? What you want is a sure thing!
- *Illness.* Do you have a medical problem, such as severe obesity or heart disease, which requires substantial and

---

Irritability If you are not at a low carbohydrate level—10 to 40 grams a day—going to that level may be the answer. If you are there and still have signs of nervousness or a "short fuse," then increase your carbohydrate level by about 30 grams a day.

Constipation Lack of potassium can also cause constipation; increase levels of such foods as beans, peas, and potatoes, both for potassium and for their vegetable fiber. Other vegetable fiber foods may also do the trick.

rapid weight control? The Crisis diet is the safest you can choose. It's this simple:

*

The Crisis Diet Ingredients: (1) Protein Powder, 60–80 percent (2) Nonfat milk (3) Morton's Lite Salt (4) Soy or walnut oil (or Essential Fatty Acid capsules). You can purchase these at any large grocery store: this is a processed food diet! For EFA capsules, you may need to go to a health food store.

Procedure: Take a glassful of milk (8 oz), with 2 Tbsp powder, $^1/_3$ tsp salt, and 1 tsp oil (or 5 EFA capsules) *three* times a day. Variations: substitute coffee for milk occasionally, or take half portions *six* times a day. For flavor, add 1 tsp cocoa or 2 tsp molasses.

Precautions: Drink at least four glasses of water a day. If constipated, increase the Lite Salt to 1 tsp per glass of milk; or take 1 tsp of Kaopectate three times a day; or add to your drink 1 tsp of acidophilus culture per glass. You may eat 1 carrot or 1 celery stalk a day, which also helps against constipation. *Do not continue this diet for more than three weeks.*

The Crisis diet is the least costly, best balanced formula you can choose. And the promise is simple: it works.

These seven adjustments should be enough to launch you safely on the Listen diet. It is designed to serve you over your lifetime—without searching for charts and graphs or burdening yourself with time-consuming recipes.

Yet in every woman's life there comes many a time when the basic rules don't apply. That's when you need a *crisis* diet. As you will see, this is also based on listening to your body.

3

Start Your Beauty Program from Within

Perhaps the best diagnostic tool a doctor has—and the simplest—is *looks.* If you look tired, pale, drawn, worried, or harried, it's probably due to more than a hard day at work or a sleepless night. And there are more specific signals of illness. Brittle fingernails with large white "moons" indicate mineral deficiencies, usually zinc and silicon. Splitting, thinning hair points to inadequate protein and B vitamins. Unhealthy gums are often the first signs of a vitamin C deficiency. Whiteness at the back of the tongue can result from stress of any kind, especially a low-grade infection. Varicose veins, far more common in women than in men, are often aggravated by a vitamin E deficiency—since this nutrient is the most effective anticlotting agent. Often, the clotting of veins within the leg forces the circulatory system to find other capillaries near the surface of the skin. Deficiencies in iron, copper, and lysine can also precipitate varicose veins. Oily skin and blemishes are frequently seen together, but the underlying cause may be deficiency of B_6 to properly regulate the oils. Skin that bruises easily points to a lack of bioflavonoids, vitamin C, and even K. When a woman has that unmistakable glow of health she may also be responding to deep feelings of satisfaction within—in short, she may be in love! As we will see, there is much more *within* us that affects every aspect of beauty.

At the supermarket checkout counters, the covers of women's magazines shout to us about beauty. But when we get to the article itself we find it's the same old cover-up: cosmetic beauty. Every woman's magazine displays the face of a beautiful model, with the latest lipstick color, the touch of eye shadow just right, the eyes widened and defined, the eyebrows raised, the hair teased over the forehead, with perhaps a "beauty mark" highlighted against an absolutely wrinkle-free face. The whites of the eyes are as milky as the perfect row of teeth. And it would be my guess that the beauty articles are much the same now as they were ten, twenty, or thirty years ago—though perhaps the range of products proffered in the advertisements grows wider each year. There are creams and lotions to smooth out "age-revealing lines," to "rejuvenate the cells of the skin," and to "nourish the neck and face." For all of these promoters of that perfect face, beauty is indeed skin-deep.

So it's no wonder that when women come to a physician with general health problems they are oblivious to the telltale signs of illness on their faces. They have been conditioned all their lives to think of beauty as something that comes out of a make-up kit. They have never read anything in a book on medicine that has anything to say about beauty. They would feel foolish asking their doctors about their dissatisfaction with their looks. Yet it's all there, as plain as the tired look on their faces: beauty comes from within. Not just the beauty of kindness or contentment or self-satisfaction, but the beauty that turns men's heads.

Call to mind the women of your acquaintance that you consider beautiful: isn't it true that it's not necessarily the one with the delicate features and high cheekbones who *endures* in your mind as the beautiful person? The model's face is recognized in an instant, on the street, or on a magazine cover. But the human eye picks up on a thousand other things after a few minutes in the presence of that face. Moving faster than a computer, the mind puts together a complete picture that even a camera can't record: the touch of redness in an eye, an incipient laugh, a hesitancy in speaking, a measured tossing of the head. Pulses and minuses are fed mercilessly and unconsciously into the mind's data bank, and out comes an impression. There is no cream or miracle lotion from a health spa in Europe that can fool that human computer.

Cosmetics: Imitators of Youth or Health?

I'm not against cosmetics. In fact, I see a relationship between cosmetics and beauty that is similar to the relationship between drugs and health. I would no more say "Throw away your cosmetics" than I would say "Throw away your drugs." But it's senseless to use drugs without first restoring your nutrition; and it's senseless to use cosmetics without first getting your body to work *for* you instead of against you.

Sociobiologists have tried to apply the analytical tools of ethology to the origin of many of our social customs. They describe, for example, how the bushy eyebrows of a (male) corporation president give him an aura of leadership, just as in prehistoric times such eyebrows shielded the eyes from the sun and so conferred an advantage on their owner. In a similar way, ethologists have tried to "get behind" the practices of women hairdressers and beauty experts—to find their roots in the survival of our ancestors.

The science of sociobiology is hardly an exact one, but it does tell us something about our desires. Ethologists speculate that women have used various forms of make-up over the centuries in a conscious or unconscious emulation of the very young. Women wished not only to look younger, but ageless. In the distant past, their very survival depended on their usefulness as young mothers, young workers, young mates.

It seems equally clear that good health was as important to our forebears as youth. What we see as signs of youth are really signs of health. Red cheeks signal rich blood and vigorous blood circulation. Bright, clear eyes imply alertness. White, intact teeth go hand in hand with mineral balance during the formative years, and are a model of the mature development of all the bodily systems. In a bygone era, youth may have been equivalent to health, but nowadays this is not so inevitable. Many women seem to grow in beauty as the years go by: they are actually growing in health. Ironically, it is now becoming evident that if cosmetics perform any function at all in imitating health they are doing it the hard way. It's easier just to *be* healthy.

Indeed, in the sophistication of beauty products now on the market we see an appeal to physical improvement rather than to visual effects. This skin cream will do wonders for you because it penetrates the cells and revitalizes them. That hormonal tonic tightens up those wrinkles because it makes the tissues more elastic. This shampoo gives your hair more body by somehow supplying the scalp with protein. In fact, many such products have a scientific basis. But there are two things that any woman should think about before succumbing to their promises: first, in many cases their effects are quite temporary, whereas the glow of health is long-lasting; and second, they are much more costly and inefficient than approaching the problem nutritionally.

The Non-cosmetic Answer to Beauty Problems

According to a study done by the U.S. Department of Agriculture, *most* women between the ages of twenty-three and fifty consume fewer than 1,500 calories a day. The Recommended Daily Allowance suggests that this is some 500 calories short of "normal." If those 1,500 calories were burned in the digestion of organ meats, green leafy vegetables, and shellfish, it's possible that such a diet would include the necessary nutrients. Judging from my own experience, however, I would estimate that only a small percentage of women on 1,500 calories a day could avoid serious deficiencies over a period of time.

We have already seen why. Anyone on the average American diet is like a four-cylinder automobile with a heavy air-conditioner to turn. Overrefined staples in our diet—white flour and sugar—not only fail to provide nutrients, but also add dead weight and make demands on the "engine" as these fuels are burned. The comfort they provide is out of proportion to their cost in the strain they put on the entire mechanism. Consider the case of a middle-aged executive secretary who came to me some years ago for psychiatric reasons—let's call her Marcy.

Marcy seemed even thinner than her 88 pounds, a good 15 pounds under a normal weight for a woman 5 feet 2 inches tall. The fearful look on her face suggested a total lack of confidence. She had been a beautiful, energetic woman, rising to the top of her profession and much admired by her colleagues and her boss. Now she was unbearably nervous and depressed. She looked worn, haggard, and depleted. She had lost her natural attractiveness.

Conscious of nutrition, she had taken a multivitamin for almost 20 years. She thought she was eating well and was sure something else was responsible for her illness. She had been hospitalized by her doctor and put on tranquilizers and antidepressant drugs. As is often the case, this cure turned out to be worse than the disease. Her restlessness got worse, her mind became dulled, and she lost interest in everything. In desperation her family brought her to me.

My physical examination revealed a pulse rate of 100 to 120 a minute and blood pressure of 135/95, sufficiently elevated to cause concern. Her tongue appeared healthy, but her gums were markedly receding (suggestive of calcium resorption) and her oral mucous membranes were quite ridged (suggestive of inadequate vitamin A).

In working with similar patients I had developed a program that met with general success, and I prescribed it here: an improved supplement, with emphasis on calcium, magnesium, chromium, other trace minerals, and vitamin C. I also set up an appointment for extensive laboratory tests for specific deficiencies. But Marcy was so agitated and discouraged by her illness that she left the lab before the tests could be completed. The stress was too much for her. I was surprised, frankly, when she returned six weeks later for a follow-up appointment, and even more surprised by her improvement! With the supplement program she had begun to feel better, gained encouragement as well as 8 pounds, and seemed brighter and more energetic.

Important symptoms remained, however: her pulse rate was still high and she had a noticeable hand tremor. I suspected the antidepressant drug, which she continued to take, had been overstimulating her. When I inquired, she told me she had doubled the normal maintenance dose out of desperation—and ignorance! Drugs do not act in the body the way nutrients do—and they are more toxic. Megadose vitamins are rarely likely to cause symptoms. Megadoses of drugs *always* do.

Ordinarily I do not change a previous medically prescribed program without first seeing some improvement in the patient from my dietary/nutrient program. And then I prefer to change only one factor at a time, so that I can isolate a cause-effect relationship. In Marcy's case, however, I felt justified in dropping the antidepressant at once. Within a week she called to say she felt much better, and that she was now able to take the lab tests. It turned out that her red cell count was still low after two months on the therapeutic vitamins and minerals I had prescribed. Her glucose tolerance test indicated she was prediabetic, probably the result of what amounted to near starvation. A computer analysis of her current diet left no doubt she needed drastic improvement in her eating habits. Hair analysis confirmed low levels of zinc (100), manganese (0.3), and iron (8). (Normal figures for these three important minerals are, respectively, 160, 0.4, and 12 ppm—parts per million.)

She responded well, both biochemically and emotionally, to continuing nutritional improvement. When she cut back on the six cups of coffee a day she usually drank, her stomach irritation went away. I suggested she avoid wheat, both in bread and cereals, and her headaches and dizziness became things of the past. Finally, I convinced her that she should try to adjust her carbohydrates. She was one of my first successes with the Listen to Your Body diet.

Marcy's concept of medicine all her life had been "one cause, one effect." So she couldn't understand how carbohydrates might be a problem, except for calories. After two days with virtually no carbohydrates she reported anxiousness and depression. Then, with her intake above 40 carbohydrates she felt better. When she stabilized at about 100, a fair amount for most women, her energy level went up and she was able to return to work in a new job. All those symptoms we call "depression"—headaches, dizziness, lack of concentration, weakness, lack of self-confidence, and fearfulness—disappeared one by one, and with them went the depression!

When she appeared for her final visit, it was mainly for a thank you and farewell. Her face was radiant; she seemed years younger. The added zinc, manganese, and iron did not have to be measured by another hair test in the laboratory. She told me that her hairdresser commented to her that her once thinning and lifeless hair had become healthy, thick, and brilliant in color. This was the "hair test" she was really interested in!

I have gone into such length on Marcy's case history because I have seen scores quite a lot like her over the years. Funny, isn't it, that we know when a person "looks sick"? Yet we don't realize that it's all a matter of degree. When we don't see obvious signs of illness, we don't make the connection that some degree of the "glow of health" is missing.

The Twilight Zone Between Radiant Good Looks and Just Being OK

When Marcel Proust wrote, "Leave the beautiful women to men with no imagination," I think he meant to emphasize how easy it is to look only skin-deep for beauty. But consider all that goes into female beauty: hair, eyes, mouth, skin—that is, mainly the face; posture, joints, muscles, weight distribution—that is, the body; and grace, alertness, disposition—that is, the mind and brain. They are all interrelated. Cosmetics and drugs seldom appeal to the imagination, but nutrition develops an entire complex of female beauty that runs deep indeed.

There are several basic facts about nutritional beauty care that we will review in a minute. First, here are some examples from my practice of how women have put specific nutrients to work for them in common beauty problems. The rule in this case is, If one thing doesn't work, try another. There is no single correlation between cause and effect when women differ so widely and when nutrients have so many diverse effects.

Hair   Whereas in men hair problems are largely a matter of heredity, namely, receding hairline and baldness, women's hair problems are either nutritional or hormonal. Because of their biochemistry, women tend to be deficient in folic acid and iron, major causes of premature grayness. Mary L., a vegetarian, complained to me of hair loss and thinning. When we analyzed her diet, we found her deficient in the amino acids methionine and lysine. After supplementation with methionine in particular her hair became full and curly. She remained a vegetarian but became conscious of the need to watch her protein sources more carefully. In her case, she was getting enough protein to avoid obvious problems, but not enough of the specific building blocks of proteins to look her best.

Eyes   In night blindness, a deficiency in vitamin A prevents the eye from adapting rapidly from bright light to darkness. There is an opposite condition called "light shock," in which one experiences pain and headaches when moving from poorly lighted areas into bright sunlight. Several patients of mine have complained of squinting and excessive blinking, and I found that they were deficient in riboflavin (B_2). Bioflavonoids, which accompany vitamin C in foods, are also helpful in a variety of eye problems. In animal studies it has been shown that cataracts correlate with low levels of both riboflavin and bioflavonoids. Bioflavonoids are known to block the effects of sorbitol, the derivative of sucrose that attacks the cells of the eye as well as the inner walls of arteries. Well-rested, alert eyes are enormously attractive. A little more attention to B_2 and the bioflavonoids can make your eyes sparkle.

Teeth   Recently I saw a report in a leading medical journal on the latest in teeth protection. Not flossing, not water picks, not painting with fluorides—but two simple biochemicals: baking soda and hydrogen peroxide. Acids that cause tooth decay can easily be kept under control by gargling with a little baking soda daily (there's nothing wrong with brushing with it, either—one of the oldest of "home remedies"). The report also mentioned the well-known fact that hydrogen peroxide protects against bacteria in the teeth and gums. I have found that Betadine, a form of iodine, applied with a Q tip works effectively against infected gums. Note that it's usually the organisms in the mouth that stain the teeth and cause bad breath. You can keep your dentist and your bacteria at bay with regular use of a simple solution of baking soda as a mouthwash, or hydrogen peroxide if you have an active infection.

Dr. D. C. Jarvis, one of the great old country doctors of New England, spent a lifetime relating the folk medicine of this part of the country to "scientific" medicine. He was one of the first to question the folly of ignoring iodine in the rush to fluoridate and chloridate everything. The law of halogen displacement states that the lower-weight halogens displace the ones of greater atomic weight; fluorine and chlorine are the lowest, iodine the heaviest. Thus, one of the effects of fluoridated water is that the body loses significant amounts of iodine. Yet iodine is essential to the proper functioning of the thyroid and the metabolism of fat, among other things. In certain parts of the country, notably the Pacific Northwest, the Great Lakes area, and New England, low concentrations of iodine in the soil make it difficult to get sufficient iodine from food alone. In those regions it is essential to use iodized salt or even to take iodine or kelp tablets. Elsewhere the common sources of iodine are seafood, radishes, asparagus, carrots, tomatoes, spinach, rhubarb, potatoes, peas, strawberries, mushrooms, bananas, cabbage, onions, and eggs.

If you have visibly infected gums, you may wish to try applying Betadine, available from your pharmacy. It works! One of my patients, a professional iceskater, suffered from gum infections for years. It was clear Karen drank a little too much wine, and relied on all sorts of mouth washes to preserve her gums and improve her breath. After I treated her for a few weeks with Betadine (in addition to nutrient supplements), her chronic gum disease cleared completely. In general she looked so much better, she told me her friends didn't even recognize her! That's how well this nutrient program worked—and that's how obvious to one's appearance the teeth and gums can be.

The mouth I have seen every variety of tongue—the beefy, red tongue that signifies an iron deficiency; the dull, smooth tongue that means low B_{12}; the smooth, sore tongue of one deficient in folic acid; the swollen tongue of hypothyroid or iodine deficiency; the magenta purple tongue of one missing B_2. We recognize "black tongue" in dogs, the telltale sign of a niacin deficiency; in humans pellagra causes a fiery red tongue. Black tongue in humans is caused by fungus. In women it is preceded by bad breath and a coated appearance, but it rarely reaches a disease state. I have seen many such problems clear up with the liberal use of the amino acid tryptophan, which converts to niacin in the body.

The corners of the mouth often begin to peel when vitamin A either is lacking or is overabundant. It was once thought that this peeling is the result of picking, but actually the peeling comes first because of poor nutrition, and the picking is only a natural "grooming instinct." The amino acids and the right amount of copper also help preserve the elasticity of the skin around the lips (more on copper in a moment). Who wants to kiss lips that are cracking and peeling? In general, there are two other nice things that keep the lips in good shape: smiling and talking! There are more things to exercise than the arms and legs, and I am quite serious about improving your whole facial cast by moving your jaw, lips, and cheeks in a conscious exercise program (especially when watching television, driving, or otherwise trapped in a boring situation).

Skin Skin responds to good nutrition perhaps more positively than any other feature of your body. And there's more to skin nutrients than the familiar zinc and vitamin A. Here are some tips I have picked up from my patients, many of whom discovered these benefits of nutrients while primarily treating themselves for something "more serious."

- Allergic "shiners" were a constant problem with one twenty-two-year-old who was otherwise a knockout. The bags under her eyes were so puffy she thought it was hereditary and would eventually require plastic surgery. She was amazed to discover that low carbohydrate–high protein levels in her Listen to Your Body diet eliminated excess water from her body—including her eyes, which went almost to normal. With nutrient supplementation, including the prostaglandin precursors (evening primrose oil—see Chapter 9), and dimethyl glycine, her allergies receded, and she no longer had that hangover look of redness around the eyes.
- Leathery skin is a problem for many women who get too much sun, but it afflicts many a shut-in, too. It's not necessary to avoid the sun, since PABA (para amino benzoic acid) is a simple protective agent. But then, we were not meant to bake like a cactus, either. Dry skin often results from excessive tanning. The antioxidants, especially vitamin E and carotene, are a natural way of preserving suppleness and moisture in the face.
- When one bruises too easily, vitamin K may be deficient—or vitamin E may be present in an overdose. If this sounds confusing, consider the fact that E prevents

clotting by several mechanisms, one of which is by interfering with the clotting action of K—thus its protective effect against heart attack. Too much E, taken in pill form, reduces clotting to the point of allowing blood to flow freely when it shouldn't: hence, a bruise. Vitamin K, by the way, is rapidly coming into its own as an all-around nutrient. It seems to have an affinity for calcium that promotes strong bones and nails.

Body   One of the first results of the Listen diet is a loss of *girth*. This is because water loss typically comes in the midsection of the body. Don't be fooled by this result in any diet—water is always the first thing to go. On the other hand, don't be discouraged if there is little weight loss and you're exercising: the muscle you are building weighs more, volume for volume, than fat. But if you're trying to get back into a size 10, the Listen diet can help you rather quickly. I have seen some 5,000 patients in the last ten years, in connection with nutrition, and I can report that the women especially have become more body-conscious even when their immediate concerns were other than *beauty*.

Behind the Beauty Tips

There are at least six things that nutrition can contribute to the beauty of the human body: (1) the growth of tissue; (2) the repair of damaged tissue; (3) the reduction of inflammation; (4) the control of allergies; (5) the protection from toxic substances; and (6) the lessening of wear and tear, especially cross-linking caused by free radicals. (Cross-linking is a biochemical process in which proteins, amino acids, and nucleic acids are altered. Some cross-linking is necessary, but excessive bonding of this kind causes skin to wrinkle, arteries to harden, and in general our bodies to become less flexible.) All of this may sound too generalized to be of practical use, but consider that I'm talking about your face, your hands and arms, your hair, teeth, gums, and nails when I say *tissue*. Nothing you put *on* your skin can do as much for it as what it is fed by. Protein is the primary food for your tissues. Keratin, whose main amino acid is cysteine, and collagen, whose main amino acids are glycine, proline, and lysine, are the main ingredients of skin. Now if you go to a health food store and buy a bottle of each of these amino acids, you'll be missing the point. There are at least 28 vitamins and minerals and many hormones and enzymes that are required to help these amino acids "feed" your tissues. Vitamin A, for example, is needed for the sulfation of collagen to produce disulfide bonds, as well as to synthesize progesterone. If the biochemistry of this intrigues you, in Appendix I you will find references for further information. My main point is that an inadequate diet, which many women cannot avoid in that constant search for slimness, is the real enemy of beauty. Women are especially deficient in folic acid, B_6, and iron. Only in recent years have we begun to understand how complex the interaction of micronutrients is, and how easily we can drift into a long-term deficiency that can damage our tissues. There is no beauty "tip" I can give you that's worth a fig—literally. A fig or an apple or a plate of good green vegetables.

Although little nutritional research is done on beauty per se, there are many studies that suggest appropriate beauty care. Consider the effect of copper on hair. This mineral is vital to bones and the regulation of cholesterol, but it can hurt hair. (Copper promotes the cross-linking of collagens, which, as we have seen, makes hair and skin less flexible.) A mineral is neither good nor bad in itself: minerals and vitamins always work in concert; minerals have different effects in different parts of the body, and different people have differing needs for minerals. So don't try to remove copper from your diet (it would be difficult even if you were a biochemist) in the interest of improving your hair. On the other hand, if you're losing great amounts of hair or if you want to restore the normal hair loss that can occur in the last trimester of a pregnancy, consider these dietary adjustments:

1. Avoid obvious sources of excessive copper, such as in drinking water, birth control pills, and cooking utensils.
2. Get adequate levels of zinc. Most supplements contain therapeutic doses of 20–50 milligrams: above the RDA, but well within the range of safety. Animal sources, especially seafood, provide zinc in its natural surroundings and thus are more likely to provide the balance of nutrients in which minerals like zinc are most effective.

3. Avoid obvious sources of other heavy metals (in addition to copper): lead, mercury, arsenic, cadmium. Again, drinking water should be watched. If your hair problems fail to improve after you have taken the precautions mentioned here, ask for a report from your water supplier or have a sample analyzed.

4. Make sure your normal choice of foods contains those with good amounts of vitamin B$_6$ (pyridoxine) and sulfur. Generally this means whole grains (for B$_6$) and eggs (for sulfur). The milling of wheat flour removes about three-quarters of the natural B$_6$ and none of this is put back in by so-called enrichment. If you avoid egg yolks in the current phobia over dietary cholesterol (more on which later), you are missing the single most important source of sulfur.

Hair growth and strength respond quite rapidly to dietary changes. Often my patients are not interested in hair at all, but they discover that as they *feed* themselves better they receive all sorts of pleasant side effects.

In the case history above I alluded to two different types of hair test: the scientific one, in which a snippet of hair from the nape of the neck is analyzed in a laboratory, and the more common one, compliments from acquaintances. The laboratory test does give valid measurements of many minerals. I am particularly familiar with this procedure because I was among the first to use it clinically more than a dozen years ago; but this test does have limitations and error. We now have other, accurate ways of assaying minerals in most parts of the body; but there is a time-tested connection between body and luster of the hair and the healthiness of the whole human being. Watch your hair more carefully; avoid excessive dyes, conditioners, tonics, and heat. Regard hair as a natural expression your self and you will find that the understanding and care of your skin, mouth, and eyes—and your total health—will fall more easily into place.

Female beauty has much to do with the skin of the face. "Milk white" was the standard among Caucasians through most of history; nowadays we admire the bronzed look, and we spend too much time in the sun. The two major causes of sagging, inelastic skin are prolonged exposure to the sun and inadequate nutrition.

Skin wrinkles with age, but wrinkles are less pronounced and not at all unpleasant if the skin retains its elasticity, opacity, and glow. Skin reacts to chemical changes, as does all other collagen or connective tissue in the body, and such changes may surprise you. For example, estrogen has been promoted for some time as a salve to maintain or restore youthful skin; in fact, for short periods of time, this hormone and related steroids such as DES (diethylstilbestrol) will cause the skin to puff up with water and fat. But it has been known since the 1930s that estrogen can cause premature loss of elasticity of the skin. In 1977, warnings were issued by the FDA against the use of estrogen as a skin treatment, but the mystique of a "hormone treatment" is difficult to dispel. Suffice it to say that DES (the anti-miscarriage drug associated with uterine cancer in the daughters of women who took the drug during their pregnancies many years ago) has most recently been promoted as a "morning after" birth control pill and as an animal fattener in the cattle business. Avoid it!

There is quite a bit more a woman can do to smooth out wrinkles than plump herself up with steroids. The female hormone progesterone has a long-term effect on the skin opposite that of estrogen: it has been shown to reverse the chemical changes that age makes in collagen. Biochemist Ray Peat argues that there is a connection between the beneficial things progesterone does in pregnancy and what it can do for aging skin:

> In pregnancy, progesterone is probably responsible for the formation of relaxin, a hormone which makes the fibrous tissues become very stretchy, so the birth canal can open without damage. Some women notice that joints become very limber for a few days each month, suggesting that relaxin can be formed even when a woman is not pregnant.

The mechanism by which progesterone has this effect is not established, but Dr. Peat suggests that—since this hormone (as well as testosterone in males) is known to normalize the autoimmune system—it prevents inelasticity and drying of skin caused by autoimmune activity. (Immune responses occur most obviously in cases like poison oak or poison ivy, in which a foreign antigen is resisted by the formation of an antibody; the resulting rash is the sign of the battle under way. But sometimes the immune system attacks the body itself—hence the name "autoimmune.")

When skin ages, the oil and sweat glands begin to thin out and become less active. This process is hastened by assaults on the skin by sun, wind, and water. Age alone is not the deciding factor; every physician sees a wide range of skin conditions at every age. The condition of the skin as far as its thickness and elasticity are concerned may also be indicative of the condition of collagen in the arteries and blood vessels. Autopsies regularly show the veins of teenagers in octagenarians, and vice versa. There is no magic by which collagen grows and remains healthy: it's in the quality of our food. And wrinkled skin is frequently the result of a consistent high-carbohydrate diet. There are simply not enough oils in such a diet to protect against drying, nor amino acids and iron to build elasticity.

So the priority of rules for skin care is this:

1. Start with the full nutritional program embodied in the Listen to Your Body diet.
2. Then take some practical precautions against the elements. Avoid frequent tanning and burning in the midday sun. If you still feel that you must tan, you can tan more easily, thus avoiding overexposure, by getting adequate vitamin B_6.
3. Take fewer baths and use an after-bath skin oil to help avoid drying skin. (A word on hygiene in a minute.)

Finally, how does a woman increase the progesterone that we've said is a key skin nutrient? There are progesterone lotions, derived from natural sources and not made synthetically, which seem to have a beneficial effect on collagen when applied to the skin regularly. But progesterone is produced quite readily in the body by a diet that contains vitamin A and niacin, as found especially in liver, eggs, and sweet potatoes—which, by the way, are also natural sources of progesterone.

Skin disorders are usually only a problem for teenagers, we are told; but in my practice many women seem to have occasional bouts with rashes and pimples. We don't really know why some young people have problems with acne and blackheads, while others keep unblemished faces. Hormonal changes are important, of course, but so is resistance to allergy and infection. Sugar and refined carbohydrates certainly aggravate skin disorders and so do excess fats, particularly rancid oils from cooking and deep frying; others pin the blame on fatty foods and oils. Carl Pfeiffer points to studies that show nearly all the vitamins playing a protective role: C to prevent acne infection, E to avoid acne scars, B_3 (niacin) to increase the blood supply to the face, B_6 to reduce the facial oiliness that predisposes one to blackheads, and A to heal and clear the skin tissue. But two remedies seem to have a more specific, direct effect on pimples: egg yolk and zinc.

The sulfur in eggs, made into a mud pack or cream, tends to shrink and reduce inflammation of pimples, especially if the face hasn't been damaged by squeezing. It's a common observation that young people are deficient in zinc, and also that a morning and evening dose of zinc clears up many skin disorders in a few days. Several studies of psoriasis have focused on an analysis of the mineral content of the outer layer of the affected skin itself, and have identified either a deficiency of zinc or an excess of copper in the skin cells. It would appear that there are common threads in the wide variety of skin disorders that can afflict women, young or old; but that our therapies must be individually devised and revised to be effective. Every over-the-counter remedy relies on one or more of the treatments suggested here, and unfortunately on some irritating drugs as well. On a television talk show not too long ago I watched a doctor demonstrate the use of beaten egg whites to tighten up the skin cells, meat tenderizer to palliate mosquito bites, and mentholated shaving cream to take the pain out of sunburn. There is at least as much science in these home remedies as in most manufactured concoctions.

Our review of skin care would not be complete without further mention of one of the most immediate reactions of a nutrient on the face: the "niacin flush." Niacin is vitamin B_3, the key nutrient deficiency in pellagra. We now assign it an RDA of 20 milligrams, and most B-complex supplements contain

20–100 milligrams. At a one-time dose of between 50 and 300 milligrams of niacin, most people experience a tingling rush of blood to their face and scalp. This "flush" occurs after a half hour or so, and lasts for another half hour. Some people find the redness in their cheeks embarrassing; others think it's simply good color. Niacin has many important uses other than this nice glow, but if you ever doubt the demonstrable effects of a simple nutrient, try a 50 or 100 milligram dose for yourself.

The niacin flush is also a good example of how clinical experience with nutrients and simple drugs can give us clues to the mechanisms of both. Several years ago I observed that the taking of aspirin prevented (or "blocked," as medical terminology would put it) the niacin flush from occurring. The mechanism of aspirin in the body, long a matter of speculation, was later linked to a new class of hormones, the prostaglandins. These hormones are a sort of pain messenger in the brain and inflammation messenger in all cells. By suppressing them, aspirin reduces pain and inflammation both. Increasing the dose of niacin eventually blocks the flush also. From these two observations I concluded that the flush reaction of niacin is related to prostaglandin activity. Individual variation in response to niacin may tell us something about the hormonal situation and might prove valuable in diagnosing a medical problem. We need more such information dealing with the elusive subject of skin care.

What we have seen in the above discussion of the hair and the skin should ring a bell or two in your own mind. If I put the nutritional "remedies" for both in tabular form, side by side, I think you will see what I mean:

For the hair	For the skin
Avoid copper, get zinc to avoid hair loss and thinning	Copper is linked to psoriasis, and zinc helps here and in acne
Get more vitamin B$_6$	B$_6$ promotes tanning of the skin and so allows many benefits of sun without overexposure
Get adequate sulfur, ideally with an egg a day for sulfur amino acids	The sulfur in egg yolk can provide relief against acne, pimples

In the following discussion of the body, you will see that zinc is also protective of stretch marks and has been known to overcome serious instances of underarm odor! The moral is not that zinc, or B_6, or eggs are miracle nutrients, but that there is an interrelationship between all parts of the body. Take care of the beauty of your hair and you will be doing things right for the rest of you. It is also becoming clear that taking care of your *brain* is the key to many aspects of beauty.

Beauty and the Brain

Biochemist Robert Benowicz wrote in early 1981: "It is a reasonable certainty that oral surgeons, periodontists, and other dental-care specialists will be the first medical professionals to adopt vitamin therapy as a routine preventative and therapeutic tool during the 1980s. The vitamin of choice will be C. . . ." He went on to cite the evidence for his bold prediction, the data on vitamin C in relation to: its prevention of tooth decay; its maintenance of healthy gums; its increase of the effectiveness of antibiotics; and its stimulation of healing processes. A short time later an important report appeared in the *Journal of the American Medical Association* for the first time there acknowledging a disease caused by a subclinical deficiency of vitamin C. (Subclinical deficiencies result in long-term problems, but do not exhibit immediate symptoms in a physician's examination.) Before this time, Medicine was reluctant to admit that vitamin C was effective except for the severe symptoms seen in full-blown clinical scurvy. The disease that is now linked to a low-level deficiency of C is . . . periodontal disease.

It had been known for years that patients with scurvy also tended to have unhealthy gums. But it was thought that vitamin C deprivation was so rare in industrialized societies that wherever scurvy did not itself exist there was little chance of injury to the tissues around the teeth because of inadequate ascorbic acid. The rationale for the RDA for vitamin C—about one-twentieth of a gram—has always been that this was sufficient to prevent scurvy. This new evidence says that we may need a lot more to prevent symptoms and diseases whose origins are more subtle than scurvy—indeed, almost every form of pollution.

Periodontal disease is a leading cause of tooth loss among adults over thirty-five. As the AMA journal report states, it has long been thought that this disease is bacterial in origin. It now appears that microorganisms attacking the gums are poorly resisted by cells marginally deficient in ascorbic acid. Antigens and other toxic substances entering the mouth are impeded from entering the underlying connective tissues in healthy individuals by the inside lining of the tissues; from another study reported in the same article, it now appears that marginal deficiency of vitamin C makes this lining more permeable. Whatever the mechanisms, it's clear that it is now quite important in preventive dentistry to measure vitamin C concentrations in the tissues of the mouth.

The control of plaque—the filmy substance that covers the teeth, supports germs, and therefore contributes to tooth decay and bad breath—is also largely a matter of good nutrition. Plaque requires sugar for its survival and growth. Plaque also develops more easily where gums are unhealthy—and we allow gums to atrophy by avoiding the foods that require us to work for our supper: nuts, grains, seeds, roots, stalks, leaves. Good tooth care means removing plaque by using dental floss; but the first line of defense is always prevention. At the same time, nutritional prevention contributes to all the things we think of as beauty in the mouth: healthy gums, bright teeth, and fresh breath. As a nation, however, we look to chemical cures for all our ills: hence fluoridation of water and the proliferation of fluoride toothpastes, about which I have strong reservations because of their long-term toxic effects on some people.

We look for chemical and drug solutions to beauty problems as readily as to health problems. Witness one of the great drug scandals of the last decade: hexachlorophene (HCP). HCP was the ultimate in disinfectants when it was synthesized and put on the market. Surgeons washed their hands in solutions of HCP. Maternity wards routinely bathed newborn babies in it to protect them against bacteria. It was added to everything from detergents to vaginal sprays. As early as 1972, however, it became apparent that HCP intoxication could be fatal and frequently lead to damage to the brain cells. The FDA put a belated ban on any over-the-counter cosmetic or drug containing more than 0.75 percent concentration of HCP. Yet cleaning agents with concentrations as high as 3 percent are still available by prescription, so long as a warning appears on the container! And we go on looking for "safer" disinfectants, in the mistaken idea that bacteria are the enemy and health and good looks consist in being bacteria-free.

Deodorants, toothpastes, scented soaps, sprays, and mouth washes probably do more harm than good, besides being costly disguises or substitutes for natural beauty aids. When we try to eliminate all bacteria we also eliminate many that are not only helpful, but *necessary,* just as when we diet too rigorously in order to appear "stylishly slender" we can easily make ourselves dangerously unhealthy and haggard-looking. A patient of mine, an airline attendant, exhibited both of these syndromes a few years ago. She came to my office for a nasty skin rash that wouldn't heal, but the problem was considerably deeper. Yes, she assured me, she took care of her nutrition—with a multivitamin tablet, it turned out. Her constant battle with weight included several days a week on a single meal, black coffee to "fill up," and large quantities of fruit juice. She was developing lumps on her neck and arms, the stress on her adrenals showed in her red eyes and whitened tongue, and she had severe stomach cramps that affected her walking. After extensive testing and a return to a normal diet, she was diagnosed with a case of sarcoid, a rare irregularity in the immune system that can be fatal. Her white-cell count went from a normal range of 5,000 to 10,000 down to 2,600 as her immune system completely broke down. Finally, on massive doses of Vitamin A she responded without hospitalization. It was only then, after she was over the worst, that she confided she had been having trouble with excessive perspiration and body odor and needed a recommendation for a stronger antibacterial soap. Instead, I suggested a zinc supplement, which took effect in a few days. I now strongly suspect that several years of disinfecting herself with all kinds of bacteriocides in an attempt to avoid body odor led to most of her medical as well as personal-appearance problems. Whenever I think of the FDA's decision to allow the popular Grecian Formula, a hair darkener, to contain significant amounts of lead, one of the most serious pollutants in our environment, I recall this case of the airline attendant and the pollutants she picked up at her drugstore.

What do periodontal disease and plague and pollutants have to do with the brain? The mind supports the body, and the nutritional input that the brain and the whole central nervous system receives provides the energy and the glow of health we perceive as beauty. We once believed that the brain was given to us for better or for worse at birth, grew to its potential, and then withered as its cells inevitably dried. Back in 1964, when students on the Berkeley campus of the University of California were rejecting the culture of the establishment, a somewhat quieter revolution was taking place in the laboratories of the physiology department. A research team of psychologists, a chemist, and an anatomist were showing that the brain can *grow* with stimulation from experience and nutrition. And not only the youthful brain, but the brain at thirty, fifty, even seventy years of age.

When neuroanatomist Marian Diamond presented the group's findings at a conference in Washington, D.C., she was met with immediate skepticism. "I showed my little diagram of the rat brain, and I stated that it can grow by from 5 to 7 percent—with experience. And this man stood up in the audience, and said, 'Young lady, that brain cannot grow!' I said: 'I'm sorry, but we have initial and replication experiments that show that it *can* grow.'" Professor Diamond has pursued this direction in brain research to this day, with special emphasis on the development of the brain in women and as adults enter very advanced ages. Her work is heartening to mothers of children suspected of having brain damage, as well as to alcoholics, to people who have suffered head injuries, and to anyone who has been told to "slow down" in his or her old age. Marian Diamond's advice on how to develop the brain is two-fold: Keep active, and maintain a healthy diet. When pressed for a specific recommendation on diet, she replies, "All the people I talked to ate an egg a day and drank milk. Do I eat eggs? Yes, I eat an egg a day."

Of course I do not mean to make a recommendation of one or two foods on the basis of one person's experience or research, no matter how intense. But many factors point to the need for good-quality protein to protect the functioning of the brain as we age. In Chapter 11, I note that our protein requirements generally lessen as we grow older; our eating habits themselves tell us this. But let's make sure we get *enough* protein, and the right nutrients for maximum brain function.

Beauty may be in the eye of the beholder, but it's equally in the eyes of the "beheld." Keep that sparkle in your eyes, those windows of your brain, and you may never want such a thing as eye shadow again.

4

A Woman's Answer to "Female Problems"

Several years ago, a doctor created a furor by suggesting that a woman would be seriously handicapped as President of the United States. During her monthly period, he argued, she might be incapacitated by cramps, depression, and anxiety, and in that two- to six-day session of every month she would be unable to deal with an international crisis. The doctor, of course, was a male. He might also have said that because testosterone, the male hormone, has been experimentally associated with aggression, the Secretary of Defense should not be a man.

The painful and often debilitating periods that many women experience are the most obvious signals of how the female body differs from the male. I have already alluded to the fact that there is a greater *biochemical* diversity among women than between men and women as a whole ("men are more like women than women are like women"). But there is a huge physiological difference between men and women. Perhaps it's so obvious we rarely give it much thought: every woman is a potential mother, and from her early teens to late middle age her body is a constantly cycling "factory," going through the motions, as it were, of reproduction—whether or not she has a baby. Monthly "periods" are a constant reminder that the menstrual cycle involves a sequence of physiological reactions in which hormone levels rise and fall in a sort of rhythm of life. The characteristic male hormone attains a level and remains there, more or less, for a lifetime. A monthly chart of the female's estrogen and progesterone looks like the Dow Jones averages and the barometer readings.

We don't really know what the relationship is between these two hormones as far as "female disorders" are concerned. For various reasons both estrogen and progesterone have been prescribed for problems in the menstrual cycle, and both have worked for some women, some of the time. As we will see, however, nutritional medicine has a good deal more to offer women than does conventional medical practice in this crucial area of the menses. To look at it another way, traditional medicine's reliance on *intervention* is the least successful here, where biochemical activity is so obviously of paramount importance. The immense *chemical* changes in a woman's (average) 28-day cycle have clearly more to do with depression and a variety of physical discomforts than does any bacterial or "mental" explanation.

Menstrual cramps are real, and for some women quite painful. Premenstrual syndrome (PMS) is real for perhaps 30 percent of the female population. Depression associated with either problem is real, as is postpartum depression. Migraine headaches are real. Water retention—edema—is real, and is a predictable accompaniment to the menstrual cycle. Yeast infections and herpes and toxic shock syndrome are real. As Lynda Madaras and Dr. Jane Patterson write in *Womancare*, "On some level it may be true that all disease has a psychological component; however, it is only in the field of gynecology, which deals with women's ailments, that medical science accepts so readily the notion that disease is psychosomatic and is so willing to ignore physical causes."

Nutrient Therapy: What It Takes

In the course of writing this book I've had many queries from women who read my first book, *Mega-Nutrition*. These questions have led me to specific research into what has euphemistically been called "female problems." The message that has come through loud and clear from these letters and telephone calls is that traditional medical practice has left them practically defenseless against a lifetime of discomfort, and worse. A message was relayed to me by a friend, for example, asking if my suggestion of vitamin C against migraine headaches was worth trying and relatively safe. I checked my files again, and found additional cases in which C was reported quite useful. I passed along the advice that 6 grams a day might prove effective within three weeks. There was certainly no risk, I said, and the cost for this little experiment was less than ten dollars.

A month later I discovered that my casual advice had virtually saved a marriage. My unknown patient was a woman who had suffered from these headaches not only during her monthly period, but for weeks on end, and recurring frequently for all her adult life. She was unable to cope with her three children; her irritability and mood swings had driven her husband away from home. She had been "treated" at two major university hospitals, and was constantly experimenting with new painkillers in addition to her chronic use of aspirin. Her diet had been mainly vegetarian, and so included good sources of ascorbate. But not until she took those 6 grams of vitamin C a day did she finally see some results. Within a few weeks she was a normal woman again, and at last report she was free of migraines even when she experienced her menstrual cramps.

There are several aspects of this little story that are quite typical of a "nutrition prescription." First, notice that I had no hesitation "prescribing" to an unknown party—for the same reason I am confident about suggesting various nutrient therapies in this book. Every magazine article or popular medical book warns the reader to consult his physician before acting on the recommendations of the author. Naturally, there is no substitute for a complete medical examination before *any* therapy is tried. Yet I gladly report what I've found to have worked—not because "it's worth a try, so why not?" but because certain nutrients *always help* and are *completely safe*. No physician could take this attitude toward a drug: drugs are *always unsafe* and *seldom* work. That's right—seldom work! One of the most effective drugs in the medical armamentarium, aspirin, is at best a palliative, that is, it may relieve some symptoms, but it never gets at the cause.

A second thing that's typical in this migraine example is the predictability of the results. In spite of the biochemical individuality of every woman, many migraines respond to megadoses of vitamin C, on the order of 6 grams a day. That's a lot of ascorbic acid, about a hundred times the RDA. In severe ailments, true megadoses are needed. This is why all those who have disparaged Dr. Pauling's work on vitamin C and the common cold have missed the point: research with doses of a gram or less are well below the amount needed to have full effect in these ailments.

Finally, the cost of nutrient therapy is usually a fraction of drug therapy. Don't even consider the fact that nutrient therapy (such as vitamin C for migraines) can be dispensed without a physician in many cases. Even megadoses of vitamins and minerals are relatively inexpensive. Most of the time nutrient therapy consists simply in choosing your foods more carefully. Unprocessed, fresh natural foods are less expensive than processed and refined foods.

There are several other symptoms of premenstrual and menstrual problems that have been identified, at least partially, as *deficiency* problems. As long ago as 1969, investigators reported in the British journal *Lancet* that birth control pills cause a depletion of vitamin B_6, which in turn causes depression. The depression disappears when adequate levels of B_6 are replaced. The symptoms of pre-menstrual syndrome are so varied—from depression, fatigue, headache, and mood swings, to swelling of the breasts, other forms of edema, backache, and (typically) lower abdominal pain—that it is not difficult to see that several nutrient deficiencies may be at fault. In some women, hormonal imbalances have been shown to be the root of the problem. In general, a better diet, and especially a low-carbohydrate intake, does relieve edema and PMS. Vitamin C supplementation, the

B-complex vitamins, and calcium and magnesium are often effective. I do not wish to imply that disorders and symptoms can be treated without a thorough nutritional analysis; it is obvious that deficiencies and imbalances of nutrients are best determined with the help of a qualified nutritional therapist.

For years we have heard the chant, "Women need extra iron." And it's true as far as it goes; but the most common deficiency is of folic acid. Low energy and depression are commonly due to the lack of this vitamin. Anemia is a clear indicator, but many cases do not show the large-sized red blood cells. These sub-clinical cases just look wan and lackluster. Enzymes and hormones depend in part on full activity of this vitamin. It must play a significant role in the epidemic of menstrual disorders. I have certainly seen cases where supplementing folic acid up to 20 milligrams per day ended symptoms entirely. And the improvement in appearance—the glow of health returns!

PMS and Male Prejudice

It's difficult for a physician to overlook the presence of menstrual cramps although it has been only 30 years since it was proved that these cramps are real cramps of the uterus. And so, for generations physicians have been down-playing what is now called premenstrual syndrome, or PMS. Only in the past decade has British researcher Dr. Katharina Dalton pioneered this field, and clinics have now been opened in the United States specifically to treat the many women who suffer from this condition. Perhaps two or three out of every ten women, mostly in their thirties, require a doctor's attention for PMS. One out of twenty women is so affected that she is unable to function for a week or longer prior to her period. It she intends to be President of the United States, she'd better get help!

PMS no doubt masqueraded as other things for all of recorded history; the general opinion of the medical textbooks has been, "She's crazy." (The word "hysteria" comes from the Greek word for "uterus.") Dr. Dalton suspected that there was a common thread in these frequently reported cases of insanity. Looking back at a biography of Queen Victoria, she noted that once a month Her Highness would give Prince Albert the fits—

shrieking at him, throwing books and dishes across the room at him, rebuffing his apologies, demanding an explanation if he kept his peace. At the onset of her period, the storm would abate. Dalton observed patients who had asthma attacks only during this premenstrual week. Others more frequently had a bloated feeling, tenderness of the breasts, and the "blues" a few days before menses. Dalton's research suggests an imbalance of estrogen-progesterone—too much of the former—and a treatment consisting of progesterone shots or suppositories. PMS is no longer thought to be something in your head.

Dr. Dalton received considerable publicity for her cause in 1980 when, as an expert witness in a manslaughter case in England, she was instrumental in convincing the court that the defendant was a victim of PMS and should be allowed a plea of diminished capacity. There is such a thing as the blues, Dalton allows. It is as frequent in men as in women, and usually is the result of rejection, disappointment, or any other failure to achieve an expected goal. But the PMS depression is quite different, combining as it does overt physical symptoms and mood swings as well as the despairing "I'm no good" and "What's the use?" feelings.

One would think, therefore, that what we are recognizing in PMS is an explanation for the fact (reported by the American Psychiatric Association in 1981) that more than twice as many women as men have at least one bout with serious depression. If one takes into account all forms of depression, serious or otherwise, then "depression" is the predominant diagnosis for women in all health care facilities except mental institutions. Not the common cold, not heart disease, not "female disorders," but depression. Yet in a publication of the American Medical Association in 1982 an article on women and depression made no mention whatsoever of PMS. The greatest vulnerability, the article stated, was among women in the postpartum period or in their middle years. "With no money for babysitters, recreation, or household help and little, if any, time for themselves, these women often have no one to turn to for financial or emotional assistance. The cause of their depression seems obvious: they are trapped in depressing lives with little hope for a brighter future."

A similar note has been sounded by feminist writers: depression is mainly a problem of our culture, our times, or even of our resistance to our times. Maggie Scarf in *Unfinished Business* and Colette Dowling in *The Cinderella Complex* present both sides of this story. As a psychiatrist during the period these women portray I must agree with their observations; but at the same time I must insist that the metabolic factor has never been given sufficient consideration. Successful women have examined their lives and their success and have found themselves to be unaccountably depressed; less successful women have examined their lives and found themselves to be *accountably* depressed. In both cases a disease has been invented, depression, to account for their feelings. In a good part of both cases I believe that nutritional deficiencies and hormonal imbalances may be the real problem. In particular, it is known that progesterone synthesis is dependent on vitamin A, a vitamin all too often deficient in women who don't eat liver, eggs, and cheese. Vegetable sources of vitamin A in the form of carotene are often ineffective, especially in case of thyroid or diabetes problems. Niacinamide is also needed for progesterone, and zinc is probably involved, too. Sub-clinical deficiencies are not rare. When progesterone is not fully active, estrogens exert their influence in an unbalanced system.

It should be emphasized that a large number of menstruating women experience the *opposite* of PMS in the week or ten days before their periods. Since no one reports feelings of euphoria to a doctor unless these feelings are related to a medical problem, we will have to consider these experiences "unsupported by scientific research" for the time being. Yet there is ample evidence that some women are more energetic, and feel *better* in the premenstrual period, as well as being unaffected by depression or swelling and tenderness at menses. Progesterone levels are normally up at this time. I believe that this result has more to do with nutritional well-being than with heredity or autosuggestion. The use of vitamin A, zinc, B_6, folic acid, and primrose oil along with the proper dietary balance has relieved premenstrual symptoms and menstrual cramps in many of my patients, some of whom had never had a normal menstrual period since puberty!

For the woman who fails to respond, the use of proges-

terone is most practical. In *Premenstrual Syndrome and Progesterone Therapy* (Year Book Medical Publishers, 1977), Katharina
Dalton gives ample theoretical and practical information—but it
must be prescribed by your doctor. The only side effect of this
hormone is a tendency to prolong the menstrual period. It is
prudent to restrict treatment to the period after ovulation and
before menstruation, roughly two weeks. In resistant cases the
dose can be increased systematically until the symptoms dis-
appear.

Progesterone has been reported to alleviate symptoms of
migraine, depression, edema, mastitis (infection of the breast,
usually during breast feeding), varicose veins, and herpes, and
to help prevent these from occurring. As in the case of vitamin
C, I share the concern of all good medical scientists about claims
of a single cure for a wide variety of apparently unrelated
illnesses. When we have unraveled the mechanisms, I am confident that the role of progesterone will be as understandable as
the activity of aspirin on the prostaglandins. We do know, however, that estrogen and progesterone are antagonists, and recently it has been found that progesterone literally displaces
estrogen from cells, preventing the irritability, water retention,
and painful swelling that otherwise occur.

Feminist writing has been profoundly aware of medical issues. Here is the real hope, I feel, of changing the prejudices
that dictate current medical practice for all of us, male and
female. In *Womancare*, as I have mentioned above, Madaras and
Patterson have made the most recent and effective assault on
the male bastion of medical wisdom. Starting with a simple goal,
making self-examination of the sexual organs feasible for the
average woman, this team has set in motion a much larger
program. Let them tell it:

> Gynecological self-exam is a sure cure for what we have come
> to call the M.D.eity syndrome. . . . Perhaps [its] most charac-
> teristic symptom . . . is the use of esoteric and incomprehen-
> sible language. A woman appearing before the M.D.eity with
> an irritating rash on her inner thighs might, for instance, be
> told that she has erythema intertrigo, for which the doctor
> might prescribe an ointment with a multisyllabic Latin name.
> This too has its purposes. Such a woman might gratefully pay

$50 or $75 to learn she had such an impressive sounding condition that could so easily be cured. But were she to visit a shirt-sleeved doctor who told her the problem was chafing . . . and that she could rub a soothing ointment on her thighs, the woman might, understandably, balk at paying $50, much less $75, for "professional services rendered."

Madaras and Patterson go on to discuss even more serious results of male medical attitudes. A now-famous 1976 report on surgery in America confirmed that the removal of the uterus, hysterectomy, was done 794,000 times in that year, killing 1,600 women. As many as 300,000 of those operations, according to this government-sponsored report, were unnecessary.

As a man, I must admit to a certain defensiveness at the anger directed at an entire profession by these and other well-qualified women. There are far too many physicians who do not fit the mold of the "M.D. eity." But radical change in any profession or in any country never comes with polite niceties. The blinders that organized medicine wears in so many areas are reason enough to campaign for change. I count it as a scandal that depression is still routinely handled in the way this anecdote exemplifies:

She confided first in her family doctor, who referred her to a psychiatrist. She was given antidepressants, and in a few weeks she began to sleep, eat, and feel better. . . . Like so many other women, she was distressed by losses and changes in her relationships: her children no longer needed her as the ever-present mother. Her husband and she had to adjust to a new childless environment. . . .

In this AMA article, no mention was made of any nutrient factor as an element of depression. Yet these were some of the symptoms of depression that we were told to look out for:

- Inability to experience any pleasure
- Loss of appetite, usually accompanied by weight loss
- Sleep disturbances . . . fatigue and lethargy
- Impaired speech, thought, and movement
- Decrease in sexual interest and activity
- Bodily complaints

Fortunately, it has not been left up to feminists alone to try to jar the medical establishment out of its lethargy. The chairman of the medical licensing committee of the State of Illinois, Dr. Robert S. Mendelsohn, put the case strongly in his book *Male Practice: How Doctors Manipulate Women.*

The first step women can take to undo this manipulation is to recognize and take charge of their uniquely female condition: the menstrual cycle. As Madaras and Patterson insist, there is often little choice in conventional medical practice between "grin and bear it" and being referred to a psychiatrist. These are the steps I recommend to avoid this trap:

1. Particularly for women over the age of twenty-five, and even for those who are menopausal, there is no substitute for a complete gynecological examination in the face of PMS or simple menstrual cramps. Even if you have suffered long and uncomplainingly, there is no need to take this as your "lot in life." There may be something here your body is trying to tell you. Pain is a signal; if you wipe out all the signals, you're closing your ears and eyes.
2. If you suspect symptoms of PMS and your regular doctor takes little note of this, ask for a referral. If this does not produce results, get in touch with any of the sources shown in the back of this book.
3. Cooperate with any nutritionally minded physician you are able to contact by giving him or her a full and honest report of your symptoms. Do not hesitate to mention any of the treatments that have been suggested here. There is no magic in nutrient therapy, but full disclosure on both sides will hasten the alleviation of your ailment.
4. Accept psychiatric help as an adjunct to medical/nutritional programs, but only after your "house is in order" nutritionally.

Ideals of Science vs. Clinical Reports

The abuses that have been routinely heaped on women by male physicians may be excused in part by ignorance on both sides.

Yet there is a certain scientific idealism inculcated in every doctor in his training in the physical sciences that goes to the other extreme of ignorance: intolerance. Doctors are intolerant of the "anecdotal report," as if it's something your aunt Minnie told your brother-in-law. Yet, as Ray Peat puts it directly, controlled scientific studies don't play much of a role in medicine as actually practiced by physicians. He cites as an example the widespread prescribing of estrogen by gynecologists, *contrary* to most of the data we have about this controversial hormone. This is the scenario he has seen:

> Millions of women with already high estrogen levels are being sold estrogen pills or injections, often prescribed as treatment for symptoms known to result from *excess* estrogen. When this treatment fails, and symptoms get worse, a tranquilizer is often added to the treatment. Surgery frequently follows. Many healthy wombs are removed as a "preventive" measure. I have talked to many women who have been ravaged by this treatment, to try to find out how their "low estrogen" had been diagnosed. They say, "by a Pap smear," or "he could tell by looking in my eyes," or something even vaguer. Only one woman I talked to actually had her blood estrogen measured.

Estrogen is known in the medical literature as a hormone that ages the collagen in skin—yet it is promoted as an anti-aging agent. A synthetic estrogen, DES, is, as we mentioned in the previous chapter, a well-known carcinogen. In the best of circumstances, there was never a possibility of a double-blind study of DES to ascertain its possible side effects. The University of Chicago actually conducted a double-blind study some 25 years ago to see if DES had significantly better results in preventing miscarriages than a placebo. Think of this for a minute. The purpose of the "double-blind" study is to prevent either the patients *or the doctors* from influencing the results by wishful thinking. But does anyone seriously believe that wishful thinking could prevent a miscarriage? The final irony is that similar studies showed the drug was virtually useless—yet it was routinely prescribed as an antimiscarriage agent for several years, well into the 1960s.

If the "wishful thinking" factor of medicine is powerful—and as a researcher into this field I know it *can* be under special circumstances—why not simply give it a good healthy discount in evaluating anecdotal accounts? That is, if a number of physicians report "immediate alleviation of menstrual cramps with progesterone therapy," why not allow for a 20, 30, or even 50 percent discount due to a good bedside relationship between the doctor and the patient? But let us not disallow clinical observations out of hand—they are still the essence of medical progress. One reason why the medical establishment might be reluctant to agree to such an "unscientific" attitude is that if the same standards were applied to *drug* therapy very few drugs would pass muster. The fact is that drug therapy is only marginally effective, while nutrient therapy typically is dramatically and decisively effective.

Once every week or so I receive little notes and sometimes extended letters from former patients; I'm sure most physicians do, but I would guess the nutritionally oriented physician is more likely to get feedback because patients still perceive his or her services as something out of the ordinary. Not all my mail is complimentary.

Lisa T. was married to a promoter, who had taken her in 15 years of marriage from a small town in the Midwest to the life of high society in a suburb of New York City. Now thirty-nine, she came to me on the recommendation of a friend, in a state of desperation. I consider her case a classic of what our culture has done to women: to keep up with the crowd she was smoking a pack and a half of cigarettes and drinking four or five gin and tonics a day; to keep to a fashion-conscious weight she was off all dairy products and "on" diet colas; to match her husband's low-fat, low-cholesterol diet she was avoiding meat, salad dressings, nuts, and eggs. Her doctor had her taking a diuretic for the fluid retention that bothered her before her period. Her menstrual cramps were so severe, even with the "new" pain-killers he had prescribed, that he had asked her to consider a hysterectomy.

At our first meeting it was evident that she had many nutrient deficiency symptoms. Her fingernails were cupped and brittle indicating an iron deficiency. (This condition is so common in women that the medical texts simply say that women tend to have more brittle nails!) Her reddened palms and irritated blood vessels suggested a chronic alcoholic state; she reported on her medical history card that she had had frequent blackouts due to drinking (many people are less honest about their alcohol consumption). She couldn't understand why she had to get up in the middle of the night two or three times to urinate. She thought she had protected her nutrition by taking a multivitamin capsule and a gram of vitamin C a day.

I ordered a range of laboratory tests at our first meeting and laid down a few simple principles:

1. Switch from diet drinks to club soda—the acid and saccharine in the diet sodas were irritating her bladder, causing frequent trips to the bathroom, and club soda is just that: soda, the opposite of acid.
2. Cut out the smoking—it disguises too much and uses up too much vitamin A and vitamin C, in addition to the long-term effects of cancer and heart disease.
3. Move up to 6 grams of vitamin C a day—just to detoxify the system from the caffeine, nicotine, alcohol, and free radicals suspected in her diet.

In a week she called to say she was better. I followed her with a repeat of the lab tests; when they were normal I began to deal with her chronic depressions. When I moved her up to 12 grams of vitamin C a day, her menstrual depression evaporated and she no longer needed a diuretic for edema. "Unbelievable!" she said. "I'm Mrs. Premenstrual and it's gone!" I explained that women in our society have been sold on a low-fat diet, because fats are high in calories (this without even considering cholesterol). As a result, women generally have deficiencies in essential fatty acids. Now, essential fatty acids are the substrate of prostaglandins, which, among other things, regulate uterine contractions. So here is another mechanism to explain why women have "twice the psychological problems of men." The next time I saw Lisa she was past midcycle and experiencing sore breasts and other premenstrual symptoms. After a shot of progesterone these symptoms were gone in six hours.

One would think that this is the happy ending, but life isn't always that simple. Encouraged by the obvious improvement in her well-being and her ability to deal with life, Lisa decided to stop smoking. Within a week, as I suspected might happen, several allergies appeared: one of the mechanisms that encourages the smoking habit is the simple fact that nicotine helps decongest the nose and suppress respiratory allergies. Flare-up of nasal congestion was traced to household mold. No one had thought to change the filter on the forced-air heater for years! Because nasal symptoms recurred quite frequently, she now agreed to undertake a simple allergy-detection procedure: a full day fast followed by the gradual introduction of a few suspect foods. The congestion was gone after the fast, but then came back unmistakably with certain foods, such as carrots and wheat bread. This was also the beginning of a Listen to Your Body diet, in which we gradually increased the carbohydrate level. Her depression and related symptoms came back at low levels of carbohydrate. When the premenstrual breast pain recurred, a progesterone in oil applied under the tongue (a most sensitive area for absorption) had almost immediate results.

At 70 grams of carbohydrate a day, she was feeling better again; then another relapse. The premenstrual symptoms were gone, but she now complained of nervousness and an inability to concentrate. She had reduced her weight to 155 pounds, but could get no lower even at 800 calories a day. Part of the reason for this impasse was that she had run out of a simple potassium supplement prescribed for her low-carbohydrate diet (Morton's Lite Salt is the most practical). Then she moved out of town. A few months later she wrote to complain about her lack of benefits. I recalled the dramatic improvements that I had observed. Why did she complain now? Clearly, partial results were not enough. What interfered? As best as I can tell: alcohol. She had never given up a drink (or two) per day, even while on low calories. Only recently have I learned that alcohol is a powerful inhibitor of the enzyme that starts linoleic acid, an essential fatty acid, on the first step to its ultimate role as a hormonal regulator, prostaglandin E_1. No way could she recover completely and lose weight and still continue to drink.

As unfortunate as this story is, it illustrates an aspect of medicine that is very close to my heart: no medicine is worthy of the name if it does not treat the whole person. "Pat on the back" medicine is available from anyone with an M.D. after his or her name. Get your prescription for the latest painkiller or tranquilizer; the total cost may be $25 for a few minutes with the doctor and $15 for the pharmacy. Nutritional medicine, or, more accurately, nutrient therapy, won't work unless all the antagonists are taken into account: poisons, lack of exercise, poor diet, metabolic imbalances, and vitamin and mineral deficiencies.

Lisa's hair test had indicated low levels of zinc, chromium, manganese, and phosphorus. I didn't know what that latter deficiency meant, but by correcting the others I was able to give Lisa her first "normal period" in two and a half years. But she was unable to remember this when she got discouraged. For my part I was glad to have the new information about prostaglandins that makes this case intelligible. This was not the first time I had received such a letter, so I was able to put aside my feelings of frustration and send her a note of advice—that it takes time and persistence to master the lessons of health—and the lifestyle habits to go with them. Since then I have learned that essential fatty acids in fish oils are even more effective than primrose oil in treating PMS. As little as 10 grams or 2 teaspoons of salmon oil a day can be protective.

Herpes, Cystitis, and Vaginal Discharge . . . and the Threshold of Medical Progress

Not since the plague-like spread of venereal disease in the nineteenth century has the public been so alarmed as it has in recent years over a sexually transmitted condition: herpes II. The subject of cover stories in national magazines, herpes is neither seriously debilitating nor fatal, but can be quite painful when it flares up in times of stress or for other little-understood reasons. It has become so dreaded because it is apparently transmitted by towels and physical contact in general, as well as by sexual contact—and, worse, it is resistant to any current medications. Various researchers have estimated that 10 to 15 percent of the population now has herpes II, and faces the dismal prospect of no cure.

Unlike the simpler herpes Type I, which is not sexually transmitted and is characterized only by cold sores (usually in the mouth, sometimes in the genital area), herpes II is an unpredictable ailment with symptoms of itching and burning on and around the genitals. These symptoms can be mitigated by warm baths, but so far the search for a penicillin-like cure has been unsuccessful. I have mentioned that nutritional treatments for herpes I are quite effective; it is also becoming evident that a similar approach to herpes II shows great promise. So there *is* hope: why then all the talk about "no cure"?

Herpes is a good example of the continuing problem of blind spots in medical vision. Consider the first major breakthrough in medical progress against plagues: vaccination. In 1769 Edward Jenner fixed on a long-held belief in folk medicine—that dairy maids were immune to smallpox because they had contracted cowpox in their daily work. Jenner developed a serum from a cowpox pustule on the arm of a dairy maid—and this is the vaccine that has virtually eliminated smallpox from our civilization. (The Latin word for cow, incidentally, is the root of "vaccination.") Yet it was years before Jenner's discovery was accepted widely, and in fact Jenner himself met with hostility and was never accepted into the Royal College of Physicians. Or consider a more recent "plague": heart disease. For years we have been told of the dangers of salt in hypertension, while the whole nutritional component of elevated blood pressure was ignored. Quite recently it has been shown that calcium-depletion may be the important factor, not excessive sodium. How long will it take for this message to reach the public? My point is that when we are on the threshold of medical progress in any disease, it is quite difficult even for professionals to accept change.

If herpes is as prevalent as many claim, perhaps both professionals and laymen alike will take more readily to the promise of treatment and cure that nutrition now offers. Cystitis, a common bladder infection, can be treated with the same general approach I have found to be effective for herpes. Follow this sequence:

1. Since herpes II seems to flare up at unexpected times, it seems quite likely that a general strengthening of one's nutrients may avoid those metabolic breakdowns that precipitate the outbreak of any disease. The first step in treating herpes, therefore, is to improve the quality of your diet and to take a therapeutic-type daily vitamin supplement.

2. When it does flare up, herpes can be treated topically with vitamin C, in the form of sodium ascorbate. Other forms of ascorbic acid may be irritating. Mix sodium ascorbate with water and apply with a cotton swab on the infected site for five or ten minutes. Vitamin E can also be applied by cutting a capsule in two and dabbing the oil on the infected area. Help repair damaged tissue as you would in other parts of the body: take vitamin A in gradually increasing doses up to 30,000 i.u. a day, and zinc in 100 mg pills up to three times a day for a week.

3. As far as a cure is concerned, anyone in medicine must be cautious, but in nutritional medicine we *do* know this: a virus can be arrested by correcting the balance of various amino acids. Arginine, in particular, favors the implantation of viruses, whereas lysine counteracts this effect according to long-term studies of virus cell cultures. Obviously, one cannot select amino acids in isolation in foods; one must buy them in health food stores. If you have done all of the above and still experience no lessening of herpes or of vaginal infections of other kinds, such as common cystitis, I recommend you take lysine in increasing doses as indicated on the label.

Recurrent cystitis usually results from inflammation of the urethra. Because women have shorter urethras, there is a greater risk of irritation and contamination. In addition to the treatment suggested above, support of the thyroid is often helpful. Concentrate on iodine-rich foods such as fish, or consult your physician about your thyroid functioning.

Finally, in the case of vaginal discharge (commonly treated with antifungal, antibiotic suppositories) consider first the measures above, especially vitamins A and C and zinc. The monilia yeast that is usually the problem here, also can be kept under control by reinforcing your natural bacteria by means of acidophilus culture. A teaspoonful in a glass of warm water is an effective douche.

The message is clear: many of women's most intimate problems are not being addressed adequately by orthodox medical thinking.

5

The Fully Sexual Woman

A touch, a kiss, a moment of fantasy can do things to the human body that no chemical can match. This is "arousal." Arousal is a process that fits in somewhere between "sexuality" on the one hand and actual physical intercourse on the other. "Sexuality" refers broadly to the characteristics of one's sex, and whether they are fully developed and expressed. Nutrition has a large part to play in all three phases of the broad human interaction we call "sex." We can deal with sexual problems more effectively if we distinguish clearly these three separate phases, noting the role of food in each.

When we hear about aphrodisiacs, for example, we frequently confuse what might arouse a woman sexually with what might help her achieve satisfaction. With this simple distinction alone we can dismiss the claims of many such potions.

It should also be clear that sexuality has more to do with good health than with what we call "sexiness." Arousal, on the other hand, seems to be associated with psychological factors—the influence of mind on body. And the sex act itself depends on specific biochemical factors, such as blood flow and the activity of certain trace elements in the glands, as well as on psychological input.

Unfortunately, medical opinion has traditionally depended on psychological explanations alone in trying to treat sexual dysfunctions. In a typical case, after obvious physical problems are ruled out, both sexual partners are examined by a counselor or psychiatrist for mental blocks. Therapy may consist of some form of consciousness-raising or even use of surrogate partners. Seldom is a big intermediate step considered: the possibility of a nutritional deficiency. In this chapter I will consider how women can use nutrients to help achieve sexual satisfaction in all phases of sex.

The Carbohydrate Factor in Lovemaking

There are a number of specific nutrients that have a demonstrable effect on sexual performance. But first I would like to consider the more general question of diet composition. Does it make any difference if one is on a low-fat, or low-protein, or low-carbohydrate formula? In the Listen to Your Body diet outlined in Chapter 2, you'll recall how the adjustment of carbohydrates results in the regulation of mood swings, and has been successful in treating anxiety, depression, listlessness, and distractedness, as well as forms of manic behavior. Because most Americans today consume high levels of carbohydrate—well above 50 percent of our total food intake—this adjustment usually is downward, with an increase in protein and fats. In more than ten years of clinical observation of the effects of this carbohydrate-lowering diet, I know that women who "feel their best" at the right carbohydrate level also report a more satisfactory sex life.

This observation is readily understandable; certainly any form of emotional upset can interfere with the delicate balance in a woman's sexual feelings. Severe depression can make sexual performance impossible; anxiety can make it undesirable. On the other hand, that "healthy as a wild animal" feeling can make a woman more desirable as well as more desiring. These are impressions that are difficult to quantify but they are amply illustrated in the vast literature on this subject.

Now, what's the evidence, beyond my clinical observations and those of other nutritionists, that diet composition affects moods? The most recent and definitive is a report from two researchers at the Department of Nutrition and Food Science at M.I.T., Drs. Hillel J. Chiel and Richard J. Wurtman, in *Science,* August 7, 1981. These researchers point out that there is ample evidence that starvation, malnutrition, dietary deficiencies, and prolonged dietary changes have an effect on learning, sleep, and "spontaneous motor activity." This latter phrase is significant: what we see as such activity in rats can be projected to human beings as undesirable "interference." In a woman, spontaneous motor activity might be any of the following: a tic, a constant worry, an obsession, a distracted state of mind, an emotional free-for-all. The M.I.T. researchers wanted to know if a simple change in diet composition, from carbohydrate to fats and protein, could also cause the "starvation reaction" in rats (and presumably in human beings). And a simple change in a *few* days.

Their unequivocal answer was yes. They write:

> The nocturnal activity patterns of rats changed significantly within three days after . . . the ratio of carbohydrate to protein was systematically varied. As the ratio increased, the rats were more continuously active . . . whether the diet contained 15 or 45 percent fat. No correlation was found between the number of calories an animal ate and its activity patterns.

In other words, carbohydrates cause more scampering around. From their evidence they argue that the mechanism of this effect lies in the ability of a high protein-to-carbohydrate ratio to limit certain transmitters of the brain. In short, the whole neural system is quieted when the carbohydrates are lower.

The relaxed state that my patients report on a lowered carbohydrate diet is consistent with this evidence. Stress of any kind—the constant ringing of the telephone, freeway driving, dealing with teenagers, worrying about one's job—is an antirelaxant. The relaxation response achieved by biofeedback and conscious avoidance of obvious stressful situations parallels our nutritional findings. The equation is: less neural activity = less stress = less interference with lovemaking. This somewhat brash conclusion has as much to do with the body as with the psyche. Here's why:

There are various systems in human physiology—the nervous system, the endocrine system, the cardiovascular system, and so on—which interact with each other to maintain a homeostatic balance. This balance is designed to preserve the functioning of the whole body, but there are obvious priorities. The brain requires a quarter of all the glucose in a well-nourished body, and it will take more than its share if the body is undernourished. The heart is obviously high on the priority list. At the very bottom of this "caste system" are the sex hormones, which are also supplied in the endocrine system. If the pituitary gland does not have the wherewithal to perform fully, it will continue to supply the cortical adrenals and the thyroid *at the expense of the sex hormones.* This "order of sacrifice," as K. J. Franklin termed it in a basic paper in 1951, means simply that a poor diet affects the sex function first.

Stress is as devastating to the physiology as a poor diet; it attacks the low man on the totem pole first. Thus that "headache" that is complained of by women who are not in the mood for sex is not an excuse. In sum, by reducing stress in its various forms a correct carbohydrate diet can improve sexual functioning and response. How important is this diet compared, for example, to psychological aspects of sexuality? I believe it is all-important. It's like making sure you have the plug in the socket before you call the TV repair service.

The Second Level of Testing for Sexual Dysfunction: Specific Foods

Some years ago a beautiful young woman was referred to me by her husband, an anesthesiologist, with an unusual complaint: sneezing and coughing without any obvious cause. She had read about the newest therapies for food allergies, and she had tried to find the culprit in her case by removing each food one by one from her diet. But her sneezing and coughing continued, usually in the chill of the night air, no matter what class of foods she eliminated from her daily regimen. She realized that sometimes one's favorite foods are the ones at fault, and that by eating more of them one manages to mask the symptoms of allergy and so perpetuate a need for them. (As we shall see in Chapter 9, this is the basis of Theron Randolph's analysis of alcoholism.)

My friend's wife was a model patient, volunteering any kind of information that might have a bearing on her problem. I analyzed carefully the many forms she filled out, including the computer diet, to unearth possible clues to her suspected allergy. Her sexual energy was quite high, as was evident in her natural exuberance and in her candid comments on her medical history. It occurred to me to inquire if her sneezing attacks coincided at all with sexual intercourse! This question may seem odd at first, but, as you will see, it is quite logical. I reasoned that women who are sexually well satisfied—as evidenced by an unabashed and joyous attitude toward sex—are also inclined to be sexually active on a regular basis. Women with high histamine levels are known to achieve orgasm easily, and orgasm quite often releases histamines, with resultant sneezing, in women with abnormally high histamine levels. (In men, it is well documented that high histamine levels correlate with excessively rapid sexual response, including the infamous premature ejaculation.) I asked her to see if there was, in fact, any apparent relationship between her sneezing attacks and sexual activity. A month and a half later she called to say that she had a variety of reactions with orgasm and that the suspected allergic reactions were the most prominent. By modifying her diet to put less emphasis on beans, salad vegetables like romaine and spinach, and orange juice, she was able to cut down on the unusually high levels of folacin, or folic acid, which is the critical supplier of histamines. Antihistamines would also have been of some effect, but as it turned out the food correction was quite sufficient. Her sex drive remained at a healthy level. It's apparent that these same foods might be considered to be mildly allergy-causing, and that the allergy mechanism may take many forms. In this case the patient probably was allergic to one of the major folacin foods, and the reaction was delayed, as is often the case.

The other side of the coin is that the woman who has difficulty having orgasm in sexual intercourse might be folacin-deficient, and thus histamine-deficient. It has been documented that histamines are a factor in male potency, as I have just mentioned; but no direct studies have been done to show a *causal* connection between observations and histaminelike reactions in females at the time of orgasm and a higher incidence of orgasm. In any case, no woman should rush out and buy the folacin-rich foods as a guarantee of sexual fulfillment. A good rule to follow is that a diet composed mainly of whole foods is going to give any normal woman sufficient nutrients for a full sex life; only in exceptional cases, where sexual problems are severe and where specific deficiencies are diagnosed, should a "food for sex" diet be prescribed.

Having said that, I can now recommend some specific nutrients a woman should be aware of, especially if she regularly has problems of achieving orgasm; this is sufficient to require a doctor's attention. First, she should realize that among researchers as well as among physicians there is a wide range of opinions on sexual matters. I have already mentioned that the prevailing emphasis is on psychological factors. Masters and Johnson, among others, also blame poor lovemaking technique for lack of satisfaction in many women. A good deal of print has been devoted to the *location* of the female orgasm: a popular self-care book for women states, "The so-called vaginal orgasm has been shown by the clinical work of Masters and Johnson to be a myth. All female orgasms are related to the clitoris." In my opinion the attempt to locate the sexual response at a precise point in the human body is to mistake stimulation for orgasm. Perhaps Freud and many psychiatrists since him were wrong in thinking that clitoral stimulation is a less "mature" part of orgasm. Sexual stimulation does so much to the body, including elevating electrical activity of the brain, enlarging the pupils of the eyes, and increasing blood pressure, that trying to pinpoint its precise components is like asking where the pleasure comes in a Beethoven symphony.

Nutrition and Libido

Once you are over these verbal hurdles, consider the nutrients that we know are necessary for *fertility*. In nature's evolutionary plan, we can surmise that what is needed for reproduction is probably also needed for the libido. In fact, we know that excessive estrogen (that is, excessive in relation to progesterone) can cause both infertility and sexual dysfunctioning. Copper seems to act in the same way. The sex researchers note that many women who have been on the Pill or who have used an IUD for any length of time report a loss of sexual interest, and an inability to reach or a diminution in intensity of orgasm. In the former case, excessive estrogen could be the cause, and in the latter excessive copper. The nutrients that counteract the undesirable effects of estrogen and copper are vitamins A, C, and E, and the minerals zinc and magnesium. The mechanisms by which each of these work are varied: since, as we have seen, estrogen places heavy demands on the liver, vitamin C's detoxifying ability is required; vitamin A is vital to the production of the sex hormones, and so helps to restore the estrogen-progesterone balance; zinc is well known as an antagonist to copper; magnesium is a powerful sedative that works against the stressful effect of estrogen; and vitamin E is another detoxifier which also increases the sex hormones.

Vitamin E has taken the brunt of criticism leveled against "sex foods," but in fact research on E has consistently shown it plays a strong role in fertility as well as in sexual capacity. Dr. Peat emphasizes the role of E in oxygen metabolism: "For certain nerve systems, both taking vitamin E and having an orgasm might be compared to taking a good deep breath."

In addition to their effects against estrogen and copper, these same nutrients produce beneficial results in other bodily functions critical to sexual performance. The thyroid, which regulates metabolism, has been the focus of research into sexual dysfunction for many years. In 1947, S. Simkins showed that massive doses of vitamin A (200,000 to 400,000 i.u. daily) could restore sexual functioning in men and women by correcting goiter problems (goiter is an enlargement of the thyroid glands because of the inability of the glands to metabolize iodine in the absence of vitamin A). One of the first symptoms of a deficiency of this vitamin is a loss of night vision; mild cases can be treated by diet alone (rutabaga, carrots, spinach, strawberries, pears, peaches, turnips). Iodine is needed for the production of various hormones, and cannot be assumed to be present in a "normal" diet. For example, the daily requirement of 150 micrograms can be met with a normal serving of fish or shellfish, but would require 2 pounds of eggs, 6 pounds of meat, 8 pounds of cereal or nuts, or 10 pounds of vegetables or fruit! As J. B. Stanbury showed in 1961, insufficient dietary iodine tends to exacerbate the slightest defects in the thyroid.

Vitamin E has perhaps the widest range of physiological effects, either suspected or proved, in human sexuality. It is needed for normal reflexes and for the functioning of the brain; as Dr. Peat has pointed out, both of these "expectancy" capabilities of the body are crucial in sexual arousal. He writes, "The expectancy process in the most uniquely human part of the brain is as essential for good sex as it is for good art or good science." Magnesium also has an effect on this so-called "ready state" through its protective role with ATP, adenosine triphosphate. ATP, along with creatine phosphate, is a chemical circulating in living things that maintains the electrical charge of living cells.

We have seen that vitamin B_6, pyridoxine, is effective in alleviating menstrual cramps and in counteracting side effects of the Pill. More recently, research has shown this vitamin is remarkably effective in helping women become fertile. Manganese was observed to be a sexual stimulant in miners exposed to toxic levels for a year or more. Many of my patients have experienced a remarkable increase of arousal and sensitivity within a few days of starting to supplement manganese. A dose of 30 to 50 milligrams is sufficient.

So you have a laundry list of possible deficiencies to consider when you take your sexual problems to your doctor: folic acid, magnesium, manganese, zinc, phosphorus (another hormonal nutrient), and vitamins A, B_6, C, and E. Dr. David Reuben, who wrote one of the first popular books on sexual techniques, has declaimed against vitamin and mineral supplements to overcome deficiencies because those nutrients are available in good measure in common foods. While this is true for those who watch their purchasing and their diets carefully, it's a dangerous attitude for anyone who has a serious problem. And in the case of sexual dysfunction, even an excellent diet is no guarantee of getting the right balance of nutrients. All the mechanisms and therapies I've presented here may seem to be intricate and unsubstantial, but in fact proper sexual functioning is no simple matter. In case after case, megadoses of the right nutrients have produced clear-cut results for my patients. On the other hand, if your sexual problems are matters of degree—of occasional disappointment or low level of sexual interest—by all means aim for a general improvement in your nutrients, starting with a carbohydrate-lowering diet and concentrating on those foods that supply good amounts of the vitamins and minerals discussed in this chapter.

The Sexual Turnoffs and Turnons

One of my patients recently told me of a conversation among several of her friends, about the status of women in our society. The eldest of the group listened with a smile to their thoughts about IUDs and tampons and male gynecologists, and finally said, "If menstruation is the curse, sex is the blessing."

Thus far I've emphasized the physiological aspect of sexuality, but I did not mean to exclude the psychological. Rather, I think psychology has been put to a very menial use in this field: as being concerned only with mental blocks or with positive fantasies. I would like to consider a much more dynamic aspect of sexual psychology, namely, how mental states not only influence but actually change our biochemistry. These are the real "turnoffs" or "turnons."

In 1967, Schilkraut and Kety reported in *Science* on a series of lengthy studies on the neurotransmitters of the brain, the catecholamines (norepinephrine and dopamine) and the indole amine, serotonin. These amines (along with such others as amphetamine) stimulate the brain; in excess they cause elation and even mania, and in deficiency, depression. What these researchers discovered is that the process can work both ways: when young children had experiences of elation or depression caused by some event, they could develop "enduring biochemical changes" in their levels of amines, which then predisposed them to corresponding mental states in their adult lives. Since then we have learned that another class of transmitters, prolactin, is an antagonist of dopamine. Dopamine seems to turn on sexual desire; prolactin turns it off.

In an interesting recent study, women were able to develop their breasts somewhat simply by practicing visual imagery. The mechanism was measurable: on thinking about their bodies in a pleasurable way, these women produced more dopamine, which in turn (over several months) aided the natural hormonal stimulation of growth of the breast. In short, although "thinking can make it so," the body is also wired rather basically to turn on and off the cycles that contribute to our survival.

What practical application can we make of this knowledge of the interrelationship of mind and body? First, good health has greater benefits than merely preventing disease. Health dispenses joy, and joy sows the seeds of good sex. The woman who does not enjoy food probably will not enjoy her body, and as a result will have trouble finding that sexual activity is hers to enjoy. There are many reasons why a woman might not enjoy food: as expressed best in the recent book *Fat Is a Feminist Issue,* by Susie Ohrbach, there are societal pressures against a woman's doing with her body what she wants. But food has also been an image of the unwanted role of homemaker, the subject of the "women's pages" in the newspaper. So the cycle has to be stopped somewhere, and the best place is at the table. By becoming food-conscious—aware of which ones are nutrient-rich and which give her the specific minerals she is likely to be deficient in as a woman—she can begin to enjoy food again.

Perhaps one way to get over certain attitudes about food is to try one of the extremes of eating—fasting. I have already pointed out that a controlled fast in an otherwise healthy person is a safe and useful experiment. Fasting may not lose weight as effectively as a very reduced intake (nutrients are needed to speed the metabolism of fat), but it does reduce the load on the entire body. A number of good studies have shown that impotence and frigidity can be reversed by brief fasting. The mechanism appears to be the simple one of lowering the stress of the digestive system to give the gonads a better share of the energy supply. Long-term fasting causes male impotence, by depriving the body of the wherewithal to produce testosterone. Similarly, endurance exercise, such as running a marathon, is a sort of "condensed starvation" that also results in a shutdown of hormone production. Both conditions are quickly reversed by proper eating. After a short fast of from two to four days, most people report the same feelings—heightened sensations, more positive moods, and especially a better appreciation of food—because of a rise in endorphins. That first meal after only water and supplements for a few days tastes like a feast. You also begin to learn what you carry around daily in your digestive tract, and what your cycle of metabolism is.

In the last dozen or more years, when women have truly taken control of their sexuality, nutrient therapy to aid them in that goal has also come of age. Let's hope that progress continues apace in both fields.

6

To Be or Not To Be, and How To Be, Pregnant

In this highly developed, scientific culture we live in we are still in the Dark Ages as far as maternity goes. Decisions about how to manage a pregnancy seem to be made by a sort of witchcraft, in which "old doctors' tales" take the place of known evidence. And the victims are not merely the disadvantaged in ghettos or rural areas, or those who receive no prenatal care in the first trimester. The victims are not always measured by the grim statistics of maternal deaths or infant mortality, but by unnecessarily stressful pregnancies and deliveries and even by underdeveloped babies. Although this chapter is primarily about preparing for birth, nutritional knowledge also offers a woman quite a bit of help concerning conception and contraception: two areas in which we are also backward for a supposedly enlightened society.

The probable outcome of a pregnancy is, after all, the major consideration in a woman's decision to avoid conception or to abort. Will she be able to care for the child? Will the child be prepared to face the world? If she is unmarried, she may wonder if she will suffer rejection by family, friends, or the child's father. Will her work or well-being be compromised in pregnancy or child-rearing?

It is not obvious that any of these questions is consciously influenced by her expectation of her health status during pregnancy and even by her expectation of her child's health. We like to think of a "to be or not to be" decision as being based purely on rational grounds: do I want a child or don't I? But surely in a woman's subconscious there are fears of "morning sickness," of the discomfort and downright frustration of carrying a child, or of the pain of giving birth. I would go beyond this to suggest that among the disadvantaged there are also subconscious fears of bringing into the world a child who doesn't have much of a chance.

To the extent that nutritional medicine can answer all these fears positively, one might conclude that I'm advocating a higher birth rate. Nothing could be further from the truth. What I do advocate, rather, is giving every potential mother the knowledge to make a completely unfettered decision. If she wants a child, even to give up to adoption, she should be assured she can be healthy during her term and that her child can get a fair start.

Orthodox medicine in this country has a pretty bad record on both of these counts. Our so-called health-delivery system is rather class-conscious: the mortality rate of mothers during delivery was four times as high among blacks as whites in 1978, the latest year for which we have official records. Infant mortality was about two to one, black compared with white babies, in the same year. The major cause of infant mortality was low weight at birth. In the United States approximately 7 percent of all babies have low weight at birth (under 2,500 grams, or about 5.5 pounds); in Japan the percentage is 5.3, and in Sweden 4.1. And mortality rates are only one way of viewing the problem. The damage done to mothers and to their babies by misguided medical advice can be estimated in general by lowered IQ and performance among school children, by behavioral problems among children that are the mark of our times, and by increasing psychiatric problems among young women—all of which, of course, are explainable in part by other aspects of our society.

Yet if we move away from statistics and look at what happens in individual cases we get a convincing picture of how modern medicine has shortchanged motherhood.

Dr. Tom Brewer and his wife, Gail Sforza Brewer, coauthors of *What Every Pregnant Woman Should Know*, are quite emphatic:

> The AMA attacks faddism . . . yet supposedly reputable obstetricians advise starvation diets for pregnant mothers. Even well-to-do women starve in the midst of plenty. It is difficult to change ideas because these errors have been taught at Harvard, Yale, Columbia, UC, USC, and UCLA; they have been institutionalized by the AMA and rigidly fixed by the drug industry.

It would not be so bad if the errors of the past were corrected in due course. But the "lose weight" theory of orthodox medicine still persists among so-called specialists in maternity. The Brewers cite a recent book authored by a professor at Harvard claiming that a pregnant woman should restrict her weight gain to 15–17 pounds.

The question of weight gain in pregnancy is a good place to start in comparing common maternity advice and nutritionally informed advice. To limit herself to a weight gain of 15–17 pounds, a pregnant woman of average weight would have to restrict her calories to about 1,000 a day. This is the level at which half of all mothers have low-birth-weight babies. Even at 1,500 to 2,500 calories a day, resulting in a gain of perhaps 30 pounds, there is a higher than normal incidence of low birthweight. Why does this weight restriction continue to be a guideline for many if not most obstetrics/gynecology specialists?

In the face of overwhelming evidence over the last 50 years about the hazards of inadequate weight gain during pregnancy, one is hard-pressed to see why doctors persist in an anti–weight gain theory. When I ask my patients why they were counseled to restrict weight during pregnancy, they usually answer vaguely that: (1) extra weight puts a strain on the body, and perhaps on the fetus; or (2) weight gain may precipitate diabetes; or (3) unrestricted eating can lead to dangerous water retention, to what is known as toxemia, to high blood pressure, and even to complications; or (4) it's hard to get around with all that weight, so it must be like any form of obesity. The assumption by experts and parents alike has been that the fetus will be fed one way or the other and that there is no connection between a mother's weight gain and her child's weight at birth. Besides, overly large babies, in excess of 9 pounds, are not necessarily healthy and may be more difficult to deliver as well as carry. All very reasonable, right? Take extra vitamins and minerals and let nature take its course.

On the contrary, all these generalizations are dangerous half-truths that don't begin to counterbalance the overriding consideration: the development of the fetus through protein. In looking for symptoms of illness, doctors have been treating pregnancy according to their only model, the disease model. They have not had sufficient nutritional training to understand the trade-off between the development of the fetus and the supposed health problems of the mother. The Brewers say that doctors are "taught that the placenta can extract protein from her blood, and that the source would be the mother's muscles. This is not true. Although there is protein in the muscles . . . it's not available to the baby." Worse yet, the potential dangers to the mother's health mentioned above—diabetes, high blood pressure (including varicose veins), and toxemia—may more likely result from sheer starvation than from a weight gain of about 50 pounds. "In pregnancy the protein demands are so great," they go on to say, "that in a matter of 2½ to 3 weeks a woman can go from good health to ill health if she begins to starve. . . . In the face of all this knowledge, doctors continue to starve mothers."

From my experience and the data I see, this sad state of affairs shows no signs of an early reversal. The figures I cited above for the 7 percent of babies of low birth-weight were from a recent government publication. But in the journal *Obstetrics-Gynecology* it was estimated that this figure rose to 10 percent in 1981, contrary to the trends in every other developed country. In the South, the figure (in 1975) was *16* percent.

A New Model for Prenatal Care

The literature on intrauterine nutrition has grown steadily in the last decade. A leading researcher in this field is Dr. Joseph

Beasley, Bard Center Fellow in Health and Nutrition and author of the authoritative Ford Foundation report, "The Impact of Nutrition on the Health of Americans." Although his interests are in developing a new health model in general (in contrast to the disease/drug model of orthodox medical practice), Dr. Beasley's background as past president of Planned Parenthood of America and field researcher for the World Health Organization has given him a unique insight into trends in prenatal care. This is how he contrasts the common prenatal regimen a woman can expect from her doctor today, and a "multifaceted, health-oriented methodology," as I would summarize them:

Objective of traditional approach: control weight gain and fluid retention so as to avoid hypertension and toxemia.
Prescription: Restrict calories to 1,500–2,500 and weight gain to 30 pounds; go on a low-salt diet; take diuretics if swelling occurs; use other medications for such things as varicose veins, tension, depression; take a prenatal vitamin/mineral supplement; continue your normal diet and exercise pattern and be aware that drugs, alcohol, smoking, and radiation can cause birth defects.

*

Objective of overall health-oriented approach: achieve maximum health for mother and thereby maximum development of baby.
Prescription: Restrict all refined carbohydrates, concentrating on fresh vegetables and fruits, and especially on protein (at least 100 grams a day); do not restrict salt; avoid diuretics, control swelling by limiting carbohydrates; avoid all medications unless clearly required; take a variety of high-nutrient supplements; concentrate on achieving the most nutritious diet possible, avoid all pollutants from the first sign of pregnancy, and undertake an exercise program that includes relaxation and stretching techniques.

The contrast between these two regimens is immense. Let's look at them in detail and see why Dr. Beasley's program makes sense:

Weight gain There are problems in weight gain and swelling, but they are not problems specific to pregnancy. The use of diuretics to control swelling results in dangerous "washing away" of minerals, especially potassium. The use of appetite suppressants such as amphetamines merely disguises genuine nutrient cravings and can weaken the metabolic system. The worst danger, as we have seen, is undernourishment and damage to the fetus. A healthy woman can rely on her appetite control center (in the hypothalamus) to regulate her intake of foods, as long as they are nutrient-rich foods. Weight gain that poses any danger to a pregnant woman is usually the result of poor nutrient density. Weight gain that results from a nutritious diet is generally self-correcting—as the needs of the fetus and the mother are satisfied.

Specifically, women who gain unnecessary weight on an aimless diet during pregnancy are merely attempting to satisfy their needs for extra protein. If protein is supplied at adequate levels (100 grams or more a day) it is unlikely that the mother-to-be will overeat. Carbohydrates are the major contributors to swelling, even though swelling takes the form of water retention.

It should also be mentioned that lowering the carbohydrate level in relation to protein will contribute to a feeling of well-being—for this is the first phase of the Listen to Your Body diet. There is no reason why a pregnant woman should not adhere to the general principles of this diet, including the adjustment of fat intake. In contrast, most women receive little or no dietary advice beyond weight restriction and taking prenatal vitamin supplements.

Nutrient requirements   There is ample evidence from animal studies, confirmed by observations of mothers in undeveloped areas of the world, that nutrient requirements increase *ten times* or more from the moment of conception to delivery. At the present time we have identified some 50 essential nutrients (even though, in the parlance of federal agencies, their exact role or optimum level in humans has not been established in many cases). A tenfold increase in nutrients requires much more than adhering to a "balanced diet" or taking the type of prenatal supplement that is popular today. Furthermore, if a woman enters pregnancy in less than peak condition, the demands on her nutrition multiply: the human body simply can't take on nutrients like motor oil in an automobile. Some cell loss is irreversible; some nutrients can be stored and some cannot.

In the last ten years we have learned so much about the increased nutrient requirements of pregnant women that the prenatal vitamin supplements sold in the mid-70s are now known to be dangerously low in many nutrients. Yet they are still on the market and continue to be prescribed. Why? Consider one item: folic acid.

Folic acid, taken in amounts two or three times the RDA, can "mask" a deficiency in vitamin B_{12}. This is because folacin and B_{12} now seem to have the same functions in general, namely, the production of the nucleic acids DNA and RNA in the nucleus of the cell. Vegetarians run the risk of B_{12} deficiency especially, because this vitamin is not found in non-animal foods. And several years can go by before such a deficiency shows clinical signs—partially because B_{12} is stored in the tissues for quite a length of time, and partially because folic acid takes over some of the functions of vitamin B_{12}. But when B_{12} is missing for an extended time, the deficiency can be quite serious: damage to the central nervous system. Recognizing this potential problem, the Food and Drug Administration has limited the amount of folic acid that can be put in a single pill to 0.4 milligrams. (Half a pound of spinach or a cup of dry soy beans provides about that amount.) The reasoning of the FDA is that if consumers are discouraged from taking folic acid they will be alerted earlier to a B_{12} deficiency, which is far more serious than a folic acid deficiency. (It takes a prescription to get a stronger pill, but why not take two?)

So far so good. But what about people who need extra folic acid, such as pregnant women? The prenatal supplements on the market today usually contain one-fourth the FDA limit, or 0.1 milligrams. This is not a meaningful amount, any physician would agree. If a woman takes such a supplement on a doctor's advice she is lulling herself into a false sense of security. Both folic acid and B_{12} are vital to her; the nucleic acids which they help produce are responsible for the division of the cell, the essence of human growth.

Other nutrients also work in close combination with each other, often in such complex ways that it is impossible to estimate exact needs. The current RDAs for pregnant women, which list 6 minerals and 10 vitamins out of the 50 or more nutrients already accounted for, show a folic acid need of 0.4

milligrams, twice the normal amount but considerably below what many women require. Pregnant women should also receive about 25 percent additional A, E, and B_6, according to the RDAs; about a third more zinc, C, riboflavin, thiamin, and B_{12}; and 50 percent more calcium and phosphorus. Their recommended protein intake is 76 grams. In my practice, I have found the minerals, vitamin A, and protein to be inadequate at these standards. No general standard, of course, is more than a guide.

Salt restriction and isolated variables The common practice among gynecologists of restricting salt intake is a good example of how the prevailing model of medical treatment fails to take into account the interactions of numerous variables. It would appear that lowering salt in the diet is beneficial to the pregnant woman: the idea is to limit the weight gain due to water retention and reduce the risks of high blood pressure and possible toxemia. All these conditions are related; toxemia, literally the presence of toxic substances, is probably caused by excessive hormone production and is characterized by symptoms of swelling, hypertension, headaches, and nausea. But it is not clear how salt reduction would alleviate symptoms due to toxemia if it did not have some direct effect on the causes of toxemia. In this model of a single or a few variables being taken into account, the nutrient value of salt is overlooked, as is the nutrient value of foods normally associated with salt.

Nevertheless, a major study of salt reduction was undertaken in 1958 to test the connection between salt and water retention/hypertension/toxemia. London obstetrician Dr. Margaret Robinson divided a volunteer group of 2,019 pregnant women into two sections, chosen at random. The first was put on a low-salt diet, the second on an increased-salt diet; no other dietary instructions were given. The results clearly favored the high-salt half: they had fewer complications of pregnancy and delivery, 60 percent fewer problems of toxemia, 66 percent fewer damaged placentas, and 50 percent fewer infant deaths than the low-salt group. Dr. Robinson concluded that salt is a necessary nutrient in pregnancy.

This may turn out to be true, but the study unfortunately could not control other dietary elements that are far more contributory than salt. At the clinic where the study was per-

98 / MEGA-NUTRITION FOR WOMEN

formed, the women were generally from low-income families. To achieve a low-salt diet they were limited to low-protein foods, since their affordable canned meats and fish were high in salt. So it is quite likely that lack of protein rather than lack of salt was the determining factor. Anyone who has ever tried to control all the factors in a diet realizes the difficulty of isolating any one constituent, let alone assuring the reliability of dietary information gathered from people in an uncontrolled environment. If we know the mechanisms involved we have a far better chance of pinpointing a cause-effect relationship. We know, for example, that salt is necessary in the blood-pumping mechanism that nourishes the placenta and thereby the fetus.

The tragedy of the Robinson study is that the protein effect on the mother and on the unborn has been reported as far back as 1935, by M. B. Strauss. Those mothers who were unlucky enough to have been chosen as part of the low-salt group lost 24 babies at birth.

A Canadian study as far back as 1959 convincingly showed the hazards of a weight gain by mothers of less than 15 pounds throughout pregnancy. There is little or no evidence that water retention in a mother-to-be is either dangerous in itself or contributory to toxemia. Recommendations against using diuretics to remove fluids have appeared in the Physician's Desk Reference for years. Until maternity cases are treated as a whole, and not as collections of various symptoms and illnesses, doctors will continue to ignore the evidence and continue to give bad advice to pregnant women. They will continue to think of nutrition as simply another type of "treatment" and not as the primary modality it is.

Women often come to me with problems in their pregnancies when their obstetricians run out of answers. It's too easy for a physician to think of pregnancy as a time of all sorts of complications, complaints, and psychogenic disorders that will go away when the baby is delivered. Jennifer S. was referred by a friend, whom I had helped with an allergy. Now in her fourth month, her complaint was quite specific: her eyelashes were falling out. She was afraid to take any vitamins other than the prenatal supplement her obstetrician prescribed, because he had warned her about "overdoses," especially of vitamins A and

D. Someone else had told her that vitamin C could cause gallstones over a period of time. Her doctor had no suggestions
about the possible cause of losing her eyelashes, but it seemed
rather indicative of *something* to her.

The supplement she had been taking for a month was one
of the better ones, but nevertheless was lacking in manganese,
copper, selenium, and chromium. It contained less than a third
of the 1,200 milligrams of calcium suggested by the RDAs—and
even that I consider to be deficient by almost a half. Apropos of
the eyelash problem, Jennifer was getting 6,000 units of vitamin
A in this pill—somewhat more than the RDA, but woefully
inadequate as a therapeutic measure. Now, vitamin A, retinol, is
essential for increased protein synthesis as well as for the production of progesterone for the placenta. Jennifer's high-
protein diet was admirable, but compromised by lack of A. The
drain of protein and progesterone could partially account for
hair loss, so although I started a program of 25,000 units of A a
day I also looked for other factors. She complained of itching
around her eyes, which suggested an allergic reaction. The only
food she was taking in extra portions was milk. By reducing her
milk intake from a quart and a half a day to a pint, and adding
eggs to compensate for the protein loss, we were able to stop the
itching within a few days and the hair loss in a week. Here was a
not unusual synthesis of allergy-reduction and nutrient
therapy. When she delivered a healthy baby boy, she remarked
that the eyelash loss was a blessing in disguise. Listen to your
body!

My message is *not* that more of every nutrient may do some
good, and little harm. My message is that every case is different
and that nutrient therapy must be based on informed and accurate diagnosis. After all we have heard about iron deficiency, it
was inevitable that orthodox medicine would begin to consider
iron the same way it deals with drugs: when a woman is pregnant, give her *iron*. It turns out, however, that many pregnant
women get adequate iron in their diets, and some metabolize it
better than do others. Drug manufacturers promote "pregnancy pills" that contain excessive amounts of iron for many
women. Iron can cause stomach upset that may account for a lot
of "morning sickness." Worst of all, iron in excess can deplete
vitamin E, thereby causing a form of anemia, the weakening of

the red blood cells. Consider: iron is routinely prescribed for anemia. But the iron in natural sources, such as red meat and whole wheat, apparently does not affect vitamin E the way synthetic iron does—and is therefore infinitely preferable. A woman should be suspicious of a pill, any pill, for which there is (1) no substitute in the diet, and (2) no specific diagnosis of need.

Contraception and Fertility

Mega-nutrition has definite application for couples who want children but have difficulty conceiving. About one of every six couples is infertile in this country. Of these, about half have a good chance of eventually having a child, since their problem is biochemical rather than a cervical or tubal blockage or complication. Male infertility accounts for about a third of all problems of conception. But both men and women can improve their chances greatly through diet and timing. We have seen some of the dietary adjustments that can contribute to greater sexual satisfaction, arguing that the same factors play a role in fertility. What we have not emphasized is the growing connection between infertility and *pollution*.

One frightening study, not corroborated by other evidence, showed recently that *functional* sterility in American men had increased from 0.5 percent to 23 percent in the last 43 years. That's an increase of 4,600 percent. Functional sterility can be caused by venereal disease as well as by injuries, so it is noteworthy that the introduction of sulfa drugs and penicillin during that period of time has not made much of an impact, or that if it has there must be a far more pervasive cause of the problem. What that cause might be was suggested by Bernard Rimland in 1980. He noted that an entire village in Italy reported a mysterious outbreak of male impotence, until it was discovered that the chickens in the area had been fed diethylstilbestrol (DES) as a fattening agent. (When the cause was identified, the cure soon followed.) That same steroid, by the way, was tested for some time in this country as a "morning after" pill.

The extent of industrial poisoning and water and air pollution in major cities in the United States is difficult to quantify.

However, we do know that lead alone has this broad-scale distribution:

- 1 milligram in food and 0.2 milligrams in beverages is ingested each week per person.
- 1.4 milligrams in automobile exhaust is breathed in each week per person.
- A *small but significant* amount of this lead is absorbed, and thereafter can only be removed by taking good amounts of zinc, vitamin C, and sulfur containing protein.

Over the years the standard medical references have revised the "acceptable" level of lead downward as more evidence of what levels can cause physiological damage is developed. Currently it is estimated that blood lead levels of 25 micrograms (a microgram is one-thousandth of a milligram) and above are dangerous for adults, and 1 microgram per year of age is the upper limit for children. Since lead poisoning is a major cause of both impotence and infertility, an antagonist of both testosterone and progesterone, it must be considered early in any diagnostic effort.

Success in avoiding conception or limiting one's family depends as much on excellent health as does success in conceiving. Most contraceptive methods, such as the Pill or an IUD, place extra demands on the body. As we have seen in the case of sexual performance, the key nutrients required here are the B vitamins in general, E, and folic acid. In spite of all the risks that have been associated with the Pill, it is still the means of choice among women under twenty in metropolitan areas. And it has recently been associated with increased protection against certain cancers. There is no assurance that mega-nutrition can mitigate any of those risks, but good eating habits and supplementation can reduce the effects of malnutrition. A woman on oral contraceptives can generally be considered malnourished.

Unfortunately, the need for effective family planning is greatest among the women who also have the poorest opportunity for good nutrition. But the problems and the blessings of pregnancy are hardly the province of any one class, race, or economic group. Every potential mother is a study of one, and deserves more than "pat on the back," by-the-book medicine.

7

Give Your Baby a Head Start

All of us receive birth announcements, some of them cleverly made up as crop reports or news stories, others in the more traditional form with a stork on the cover holding a pink or blue blanket. Among the ones I receive there is frequently a personal note from the mother. This, for me, is "How the story came out." A recent note concluded:

> He is such a beautiful baby. I can't believe he's real. To think that a year ago I had given up hope, and four months ago I wished I *had* given up hope. . . . I have never felt better in my life, and I can't imagine if I ever will! Thank you for being on my side through it all. You've given me a big, beautiful, wonderful world!

As welcome as such a note is, it typifies a lingering problem in all forms of medicine that only nutritional medicine seems to be doing anything about: too much thanks to the doctor. In the case of childbirth, especially natural childbirth, in which the mother remains an active participant throughout labor and delivery, it seems quite ironic that the mother should not take full credit for the miracle of birth. There should be a sense of partnership between physician and patient. But when a healthy child is born, a mother has every reason to feel that *she* is the one who created this wonderful new world. By the same token, she must take the major responsibility for the condition in which the new baby sets out on his or her journey.

As we have seen, a weight at birth of more than 5½ pounds is a critical factor in the health of the newborn. Most women have control over this aspect of pregnancy. It also appears that complications at birth are directly related to birth-weight and prenatal nutrition. Here again the mother must take most of the responsibility. Heredity, preexisting medical problems, and various degrees of birth defects are beyond her control. But by applying sound nutritional principles in pregnancy and the first few years of life a mother can increase the chances greatly of giving her child a head start. Let's examine the evidence.

Neuropsychiatric Disorders: When Do They Begin?

Dr. Douglas Shanklin recently published a summary of eight studies of the most common disorders of the newborn, in relation to neurological problems later in life. In all, more than 3,200 children, divided into study groups and control groups, were followed in these studies. The least correlation between low weight at birth and the development of a problem was in the case of behavioral disorders: close to 9 percent of the low-birth-weight children developed behavioral disorders. Yet in the group of children who had weighed more than 5½ pounds at birth only 2.8 percent developed similar problems. That is, when birth-weight was normal behavioral problems were less than a third of those of low-birth-weight babies.

Statistics such as these can often be misunderstood and are seldom exciting. But the numbers of infants involved were such that significant correlations were discovered in cerebral palsy, epilepsy, hearing disorders, mental deficiency, reading disorders, and eye coordination disorders. And the correlations were high—that is, low birth-weight could be presumed to be a prominent cause of these disorders—in 12 to 22 percent of the cases. In the case of autism, the only available study involved only 50 babies, and the resulting correlation with low birth-weight was positive but not statistically significant. A similar pattern was observed in complications of pregnancy as causes of neurological disorders. Here there was even a stronger causal relationship (more than 50 percent in the case of autism). Without going into further details, I think it's safe to say that neuropsychiatric problems begin very early in life indeed. And proper maternal care has a lot to do with preventing them. Some experts estimate that half of these disorders are preventable.

The newly developed field of amniocentesis, in which metabolic and genetic abnormalities can be detected in the uterus, has received much attention as a means of prevention. For the abnormalities that can be detected through amniocentesis, however, prevention consists of induced abortion; and the types of defects this method can diagnose form only a fraction of all types of birth defects and mental retardation. It's not clear if any of the defects that can be predicted by amniocentesis could have been prevented by excellent nutrition on the part of the mother before and immediately after conception. It seems likely that many could. We know what terrible power drugs have on the fetus, ever since thalidomide.

If any doubt remains about the critical nature of weight at birth, it should be dispelled by the voluminous studies done abroad, mainly since and during World War II (large populations during the latter period suffered enforced malnutrition of mothers). In any scientific analysis, a compelling factor is the corresponding rise of two variables. Here, for example, as the birth-weight decreases so does the mental health of the infant. In one study in 1975, children with birth-weights at the abnormally low level of 3 pounds were followed for a five-year period. Nine out of ten had IQs under 100; seven out of ten had behavior problems; five out of ten had physical defects.

The Vulnerable Brain

The brain develops rapidly, in surges, from gestation to the third year. Moreover, it maintains a sequence in which its highly complex functions are put into place at precisely the right moments. If the brain suffers from malnutrition at an early stage, in general this cannot be corrected at a later stage. Prenatal brain damage, for example, seems to be irreversible, whereas early malnutrition from birth to a year or so can be overcome by increased attention to diet, without apparent disruption of brain development.

The rapid growth of the brain is a necessity, a blessing, and, at the same time, the reason for its vulnerability. The entire central nervous system must grow to its full potential quickly to be able to control the intricate mechanisms of the eyes, ears, sense of touch and smell, circulatory system, and heart. Recent research has shown that the fetus is more sensitive to a wider range of external influences than we ever dreamed of. Not only does the fetus listen to music and voices, and react favorably or unfavorably to either; it also can sense subtle changes in its mother's moods. Provocative studies have indicated that un-born babies "know" they have been unwanted even if their mothers are not fully aware of this fact themselves. After birth they show this feeling of rejection by turning away from the breasts of their mothers, at the same time accepting milk from strangers. One wonders if the fetus cannot also sense a lack of proper nourishment, and "bang the dish" in the womb.

In any case, even though the fetal brain takes nutrients for itself first in the normal order of primacy, it bears the brunt of deficiencies. Advanced sensing mechanisms have been able to monitor the growth patterns of the brain, as a result of which we now know that malnutrition does not primarily affect the *structure* of the brain but rather its *interrelationships*. Without the protein building blocks, the amino acids, in sufficient numbers, the brain sacrifices its "transmission lines" first. Then the hor-mones in the pituitary gland, which regulates physical growth among other things, are reduced. Thus low-birth-weight babies also tend to be underweight and undersize, though, of course, the reverse is hardly true. Finally the brain cells themselves stop replicating. Without sufficient mass and density in the formative years (up to age three), the brain has little chance of growing thereafter.

What is brain food? Protein and essential fatty acids. Both occur in greater amounts when carbohydrates are lowered. This is why the Listen to Your Body diet is also good for your unborn baby. If you take care of the brain, the brain will take care of the body. Here are some specific ideas about prenatal menu planning, adapted from the Listen diet:

1. Rely on eggs as your basic protein source. Eat them at any time of the day, but try to make them the first item on your menu. Avoid overcooking eggs. A burnt egg is harder to digest and has lost a lot of its proteins. Don't separate the yolk from the white and eat only the white—that's not where the protein is, mainly. In fact, don't try to separate any natural food; all the components of a food were designed to work synergystically. If you're concerned about cholesterol intake, chop a little onion and sauté it with your eggs to facilitate the excretion of animal fats. Eggs can also be taken raw in a blender drink.

2. Eat protein foods as snacks: bits of fish, lean meat, sardines from a can, tuna and mayonnaise on crackers or as a raw vegetable dip. This way you'll avoid carbohydrate snacks, which tend to be an amalgam of salt, sugar, and empty cellulose. Don't go overboard on trimming the fat off meat and draining the sardines. Fat is *not* a dirty word. You won't desire fatty foods if you avoid the starchy foods that tend to sop up the fat. Snacks are a good way to eat all your meals; there's no law, dietary or otherwise, that says you have to eat many things at one sitting.

3. Get plenty of whole milk, unless you have a milk allergy. Again, raw milk, if available, would be best; but there's no reason to avoid pasteurized whole milk during pregnancy. Skim milk is an unnecessary fad at such a time.

4. When you eat grains, get the best available. That means whole wheat, wheat germ as a cereal (refrigerate it), and even such innocent grain as popcorn—buttered if you prefer. (A reasonable amount of butter with any grain is natural and pleasant.) Eat plenty of fiber.

5. Don't expect too much nourishment from salads—unless you include plenty of the leaves that are more difficult to shop for and prepare: spinach, kale, swiss chard. Let the greenness of the leaf be your guide to nutrient density.

6. In addition to grains and tubers, the food type to watch to keep your carbohydrates down is beans. Beans are a good source of protein, of course, but they also contribute heavily to your carbohydrate total. Peas are in this

category, green beans somewhat, and most other vegetables not at all. Even an avocado half is a reasonable
source of food variety on this low-carbohydrate regimen.
7. Eat for two—literally. Spend more on yourself, but only
if it doesn't come in a can or a package. Then keep
cooking to a minimum.

These guidelines are simple enough to remember when you
shop and when you don't have time or room for a menu guide
in your kitchen. There is one further hint for the pregnant
eater that requires a little more information.

Soybeans are renowned for their protein, and so one would
think they are a good alternative for a mother-to-be—especially
if she is a vegetarian or if her budget is tight. Recently there
have been some studies, however, which suggest that soy causes
problems in the absorption of iron. A federally sponsored University of Kansas project showed that when textured soy flour
was mixed with hamburger, iron absorption was less than half
that of hamburger alone. As I have mentioned, iron deficiencies
have been oversold to the American public relative to other
mineral deficiencies. Yet this is a serious implication—if not for
the United States, certainly for countries without our animal-
protein sources. But it is not entirely unexpected. Soy seems to
have an effect on zinc as well.

Several of my patients, in fact, have apparently suffered a
deficiency in zinc caused by soy in the diet. One of them, Maureen F., came to me early in her first pregnancy, suffering from
bouts of anxiety. After a few weeks on a carbohydrate-
regulating diet, she seemed at her best at about 35 grams of
carbohydrate a day. I thought that this alone, a considerable
drop from her previous intake, might explain her symptoms.
But then her mineral assay revealed a very low zinc level. Supplementation failed to bring the level up to normal. The only
possibility was malabsorption—and I suspected her high soybean intake. Maureen had been a vegetarian off and on for
many years and had shown no signs of deficiency. But now, with
the additional demands of her pregnancy, the lack of zinc had
become dangerous. With a change in protein sources her zinc
levels returned to normal. Maureen is also one of my "grad-

uates" who write from time to time to tell me how much the carbohydrate-regulating diet has helped them.

Breast Feeding and the Blues

There is not a shadow of a doubt—though styles may change and fads may come and go—that breast feeding is ideal for infants. Some mothers have the patience and the time to nurse their babies for a year or a year and a half. Six months, however, is normally adequate to obtain the major benefits of mother's milk, which are:

1. *Early immunity from infections and disease.* The colostrum or "first milk" that a mother's breast feeds her baby in the first few days after birth contains a whole range of immune substances (immunoglobins) that protect the infant from such things as polio, influenza, staph infections, and viruses. In addition, if the child picks up a foreign substance of some kind, in nursing he passes it to his mother, who develops an antibody against it.
2. *Easy digestibility.* Synthetic formulas or cow's milk cannot match the digestibility of mother's milk. The prevailing opinion in many medical circles that substitutes are "just as good" is typical of their attitude about such "minor" things as digestibility.
3. *Close contact between mother and child.* The psychological aspects of feeding are likewise ignored by doctors who can only appreciate convenience and avoidance of extra work. Nursing is difficult for many young mothers, and sometimes psychologically demanding. But with our new knowledge of the interaction of mother and child *before* birth we should be able to appreciate how vital this is after birth.

Breast feeding is on the upswing in the United States. After a steady decline to 18 percent in 1966, by 1978 some 45 percent of mothers chose to nurse their babies in infancy. Since this is the only source of nutrients for about six months, a vital period of brain development, it is particularly significant that the amino acid delivery of mother's milk is far superior to anything that can be duplicated synthetically. Iron and zinc are also well absorbed, and the fatty acids and cholesterol in mother's milk are better suited to the baby's metabolism than substitutes.

There was once some opinion that the strain on the young mother in attempting to nurse at all hours was part of the "postpartum blues" syndrome, and hence a reason for using formula instead. Carl Pfeiffer quotes an observer writing in the year 1820:

> It is well known that some women, who are perfectly sane at all other times, become deranged after delivery, and that this form of disease is called puerperal insanity. . . . The most common time for the disease to begin is a few days, or a few weeks, after delivery; sometimes it happens after several months, during nursing, or soon after weaning. The approach of the disease is announced by symptoms which excite little apprehension because they so often occur without any such termination. . . . her conduct and language become wild and incoherent, and at length she becomes decidedly maniacal; it is fortunate if she does not attempt her life before the nature of the malady is discovered.

Pfeiffer suggests that this form of depression, which is still routinely treated today as of psychogenic origin, has something to do with the high levels of copper which are reached during pregnancy and which do not abate for several months after delivery. Noting that postpartum psychosis occurs much more frequently after the birth of a male, he rules out the possibility of estrogen's being the cause, since higher levels of estrogen remain in a woman's body after the birth of a female. Note that "puerperal" is derived from the Latin word for "boy."

It is obvious that a mother who is unable to function properly cannot feed her baby, whether she nurses or not. Since the incidence of this form of "insanity" is still quite high, I consider it a challenge to nutritional medicine to formulate a research model to test several possibilities. Nutrient depletion from the trauma of childbirth is one area of investigation. Copper poisoning, as Pfeiffer suggests, is another. Is breast feeding, or rather lack of it, yet another factor? Or are all of these and possibly other nutrient or pollution factors to be considered as a whole?

The First Three Years

When the baby is ready for solid foods, usually not earlier than four months nor later than six, the role of nutritional medicine takes another turn. This is the period when mothers are most sensitive to all sorts of advice. Are vitamin/mineral supplements necessary? What about prepared baby food versus properly mixed food from the home table? Some critics claim that iron is the only mineral or vitamin (unless the baby seldom sees sunlight) that must be supplemented. If the baby is born prematurely, of course, a complete supplement must be given.

A mother must rely on the advice of her pediatrician, but she can never go wrong by remembering the principles that got her this far. First, protein remains the number one nutrient—the brain food. The baby may appear to be developing only his or her reflexes, lungs, and smile, but the completion of the brain is the fundamental task at hand. To get adequate protein after the baby is weaned, whole food from the family table, mashed in a blender, is no doubt superior to anything you can take off a supermarket shelf. Even though the baby food companies have mended their ways and taken some of the sugar and salt out of their products, there's no reason why you can't do better. Second, pollution and poisoning remain the number one worry. The number of things a toddler can get his or her hands on defies the imagination. Lead is still a common ingredient of many manufactured items. It is simple common sense to get a toxic-metals assay, either via a hair test or otherwise, if your infant shows any signs of colic or hyperactivity. If your pediatrician pooh-poohs the idea, find another pediatrician.

Even as you give your child the benefits of preventive medicine, you are also passing on good eating habits—perhaps subconsciously, but very positively. Your careful selection of foods can easily establish your child's eating habits for a lifetime—and good eating habits are the most precious "silver spoon" you can provide.

8

Feed Your Family Better and for Less

A mother of four young boys remarked to me once that she was the best-fed woman she knew because she ate only what her kids left on their plates. For similar reasons, I find that leftovers are usually the most nutritious things in the refrigerator. People who don't eat potato skins and the fine white tissue that surrounds the sections of an orange are spendthrifts. We search the world for delicacies to munch on, and scorn the watermelon seed. (Instead of scraping them into the garbage pail, you can crunch on them as you eat the melon, or use them to make a delicious snack: rinse briefly, place on a cookie sheet for a few minutes in a 350° oven, salt, and serve warm or save as a low-carbohydrate alternative to chips or crackers. Use your imagination to create your own snacks—see recommended books in Appendix I.) And the nutrients that slip away in cooking and freezing could feed a small country. Little by little Americans have moved away from "food sense" until today we consider one of our greatest national accomplishments to be the range of products on supermarket shelves.

To a great extent the dominance of "shelf shopping" in our habits is the result of male thinking dictating female behavior.

It was male thinking that convinced women they would be happier if they could shop once a week, in one place. It was male thinking that talked them into the freezer in the garage. It was male thinking that blessed the convenience food as a time-saver for the harried housewife or the career woman. And it still is male thinking—marketing executives and the advocates of a permissive society—that tells women their families are best left to their own devices in choosing what they want to eat. Hence, the leftovers and unfinished plates.

The person who shops and cooks for a household—and nine times out of ten it's still a woman, in spite of so-called role reversals—has a difficult dilemma to contend with. And she typically solves it by compromising. Here are some of the pros and cons she must weigh:

Frozen or fresh? Vegetables that have been stored for long periods of time lose many nutrients, we are told; so why not buy frozen vegetables, whose vitamins are locked in if they are blanched properly? Lettuce, for example, can be kept for weeks if it is moist. Research by Cheraskin and others has shown how many fruits and vegetables are stored in warehouses for months before they find their way to the produce section of your supermarket. The water-soluble vitamins such as C are particularly fragile. On the other hand, fresh vegetables are a known quantity much of the time, especially if you shop at a farmer's market or a produce store that's well known to you. You can also improve your chances by buying produce in season, inspecting everything closely for signs of aging, and shopping often, ideally just for the day's needs.

Boiled, fried or steamed? Tubers and roots, such as potatoes and carrots, require cooking, either to be edible or to release their nutrients in a digestible form. Almost all other vegetables are frequently eaten raw, but they are easier to digest for most people in cooked form. To avoid unnecessary nutrient losses, use as little water as possible in heating frozen vegetables and use a simple vegetable steamer to hold fresh vegetables over boiling water in a saucepan. Washing rather than scraping or peeling vegetables saves the nutrient-rich outside layers of vegetables. Canned vegetables are the poorest sources of nutrients to begin with, and are further damaged if not carefully warmed rather than boiled. Most nutritionists warn us against fried foods, because of the fat; before we come to this issue, we should at least recognize that quick-fried vegetables are relatively nutrient-protected. Stir-fried Chinese vegetables or deep-fried Japanese vegetables and seafood are good examples of nutrient-sparing cooking.

Convenience foods or from-scratch? There is no question that anyone can make a better pizza, taco, burrito, or complete dinner than can be found in frozen form. The question is time and cost. It's much faster to heat up a TV dinner for one person, and certainly a lot cheaper, than cooking a small portion of meat, potatoes, and vegetable. The alternative is to plan two or three meals in advance and make creative use of leftovers. Even a homemade meatloaf, trotted out of the refrigerator for sandwiches one day and as a main dish the next, is better nutritionally than any boxed, canned, or foil-wrapped imitation. *All fresh foods have many uses.*

Condiments or natural flavorings? There is so much salt and sugar in processed foods that this alone is enough to condemn their widespread use. If one is on a non-processed-food diet, normal amounts of table salt pose no problem. It is the high ratio of sodium to potassium that causes the problem, not salt in itself. For example, virtually all vegetables and grains contain ample potassium and low sodium, but most processed foods (and dairy foods) are just the opposite. Morton's Lite Salt is a potassium-rich alternative at little extra cost. In place of catsup, which is heavy with sugar and corn sweeteners, try to use herbs, garlic, or onions for spice, with tomato paste if the tomato flavor is called for. Even spaghetti sauce contains a lot of sugar; is the slight convenience of opening a can or jar worth that extra dose of sucrose? Taco sauce is made from tomatoes, has much more flavor than catsup, and contains no sweeteners. In addition to avoiding sugar, one can also avoid packaged condiments altogether by grating or chopping raw vegetables to go along with the usual spices and sauces.

Fruits, fruit juices, flavored drinks, or colas? It's not so clear that fruit juices are the reasonable alternative to colas and watered-down juice drinks. Certainly they are better, but they too contain large amounts of sugar. Because of the idea that "fresh fruits and vegetables" are good nutrition, we may run to the conclusion that we can eat all the fruits we want. The actual fruit is best, because it offers fiber as well as the bioflavonoids and water-soluble vitamins, but more than two apples, pears, or oranges a day is usually excessive. Mineral water or plain soda water, either alone or blended with portions of fruit, is a pleasant substitute for cola drinks.

Breakfast cereals, fortified or not? Granola and "natural" cereal products are criticized for substituting honey for sucrose and then slapping a "fancy" price on the bag. The major cereal manufacturers claim that there's no more sugar in one of their servings than in an apple or orange—and that may also be true. William Rusher defends the makers of breakfast candy on the grounds that at least it gets the kids to eat something, and something is better than nothing. On the other side of the political battle line, consumer advocates claim that some cereals contain too much vitamin A and D. Is plain wheat germ the answer? The elimination of as much sugar as possible should be the guideline—including the sugar added at the table. In the blandest of cereals, berries, raisins, or fruit slices are much more acceptable than sugar. The next step is to find the least-processed of cereals. And don't neglect cooked cereal, preferably regular instead of instant.

Butter or margarine, whole or skim milk? This is the touchiest question of all, and it requires a full answer in connection with heart disease. It should be noted here that nutrition information that the homemaker is likely to get in newspaper columns on the risk of cholesterol may seem to be overwhelming, but it's largely a matter of repeating some rather limited research data. A recent popular book suggests, under the title "How to Get Reliable Nutrition Advice," that one of the best sources is a registered dietitian. It turns out, however, that a registered dietician need only complete a college course of study in dietetics and intern at a hospital to earn this distinction. On the other hand, the author dismisses as "unschooled quacks" and "self-styled nutritionists" the many biochemists, doctors, and researchers who actually work in the field. Dietitians repeat pronouncements from such organizations as the Center for Science in the Public Interest, which repeats statements from the American Heart Association, which repeats the results of a few studies—and butter is declared dangerous! As we will see, the milk question is not open and shut, either. Read on.

Junk Food or Junked Food?

The seven issues I have raised above have both a theoretical and a practical side. They weigh heavily on women because mothers are the ones who must make the daily choices about food. Women usually have to rationalize their choices to their families, too; it is not enough just to call something "junk food" and make it stick. I find that the simplest way to separate the issues is to make it clear what we're talking about. What is a junk food? A processed food? A whole food? A nutrient-dense food? And what are the foods I have called "junked"?

Jeffrey Bland, professor of nutritional biochemistry at the University of Puget Sound and director of the Bellevue-Redmond Medical Laboratory in Bellevue, Washington, is one of the leading exponents of nutrient therapy in this country. He recently reported, in *Psychology Today,* on the very real effects of junk food. His is biological medicine at its best, in stark contrast to the conception that we see in a recent nutrition book presenting the view of dieticians:

> Ethical, well-trained nutritionists do not recommend an array of expensive vitamin, mineral, or protein supplements since the nutritional needs of nearly all people can be met through the diet. . . . Spurious diagnoses [like] adrenal insufficiency [or] hypoglycemia . . . can rarely be confirmed by appropriate medical tests performed by physicians without a vested interest in some dietary scheme.

A pediatrician referred a twelve-year-old boy to Dr. Bland's laboratory for a nutritional evaluation. The boy had constant stomach pains, fatigue, and recurring bad dreams. Showing little self-control, he had become increasingly aggressive at school, yet had no overt medical problems, and his symptoms differed from those of hyperactivity. A diet analysis showed a classic junk-food syndrome of sugared cereal, chocolate milk, soft drinks, and desserts, and blood tests showed a corresponding deficiency in B vitamins. Not only were foods rich in the B vitamins missing from his diet, but the sugary foods put further burdens on the same vitamins to metabolize sucrose. After three weeks of B-complex vitamin supplements and a solid diet of nutrient-rich foods, the deficiencies disappeared. His aggressive behavior was noticeably reduced and his schoolwork improved.

The link between junk foods and aggression has been explored by psychiatrist José Yaryura-Tobias, research director of the North Nassau Mental Health Center in Manhassett, New York, and by clinical biochemist Raymond Shamberger and pediatrician Derrick Lonsdale of the Cleveland Clinic. In both cases, patients whose violent behavior was inexplicable by conventional medical diagnosis were found to be deficient in one or more B vitamins, notably B_1, B_3, and B_6. Symptoms took slightly different forms, but heavy amounts of sucrose were typical in the diets of all the patients. Dr. Bland explains that the brain is disturbed in such cases in two ways—by "metabolic debris" that has failed to convert to usable energy because of a lack of enabling vitamins, and by the loss of energy. He says, "Junk food has, of course, been blamed for all manner of ills. The new evidence does show that without a proper ratio between key vitamins and minerals on the one hand and calories on the other, brain function and behavior may be disturbed."

Junk food is, then, "empty calories," primarily sucrose. In contrast, we often refer to fast food in general by this name. Yet the tacos, the french fries, and even the hamburgers with their refined-white-flour buns all have redeeming nutritional features. Most of all, it's the unrelieved consistency of such a diet that's the basic problem. Sugar-laden foods such as ice cream, doughnuts, cake, milkshakes, and colas are hardly foods at all, and if taken in sufficient amounts over a prolonged period of time can cause a number of deficiencies. A vitamin B deficiency may not be the first deficiency to appear, and if it does it may have other undesirable metabolic effects than the disturbances of the brain we have seen above.

Processed foods are, of course, a much larger category than junk food, and there is nothing intrinsic in processing that makes them nutritionally poor. A vitamin pill is, in fact, a processed food. By freezing strawberries the food industry can deliver a nutritious food to your table in its off-season. By synthesizing vitamins and minerals the drug industry can deliver megadoses of nutrients to your body that foods alone cannot supply. Processing can be as light as the wax on an apple or as heavy as artificial whipped cream in an aerosol can. So as a general rule processing is only as bad as the distance it removes food from its natural state. We have become so accustomed to "manmade" foods, however, that we easily forget this simple rule and don't even realize that a food is processed. I have met young people who think that an actual tuna fish is a little strange outside a can, or that peas taste more natural when they come from the shelf and not from the pod. Bread is processed to varying degrees; as we have seen, the most serious kind of processing is that which is done not for the benefit of the product or the consumer but for the convenience and profit of the manufacturer—in this case, the removal of the wheat germ and bran in milling.

Many processed foods are quite close to the natural state from which they came. Cheese, yogurt and butter are protected from spoilage by the simple, age-old processes that convert them from milk, with little loss of nutrients. Oils are pressed from corn, olives, soy beans, and numerous other foodstuffs; it is only when high-temperature pressing, common nowadays in vegetable oils, is used that serious nutrient losses occur. It is when processing involves the addition of various things together to create a product that one must be wary. Thus, a can of sardines can more readily be accepted than canned ravioli in meat sauce. A good rule for nutritionists is, "Eat only living things." That is, eat only things that were alive before they were harvested and taken to the store: vegetables, fruit, eggs, grains, meat, and fish. It's clear that there is no easy guideline, except to look for the least-tampered-with food. What we have to worry about in particular is chemical tampering: pesticides, preservatives, and cosmetic tricks.

The pasteurization of milk is a prominent example of food

tampering that has been accepted as dogma in most of Western society. There is a vast body of evidence on both sides of the issue, but the reality is that very few people have a choice. In this country raw milk is available only in parts of California, to my knowledge. The case for pasteurization is simply the control of microorganisms and spread of disease. But the use of milk as a beverage has been promoted to such an extent that it can be legitimately asked if we are not doing greater harm to those who are lactose-intolerant. Medical columnist Dr. Lawrence Lamb estimates that one in four people in the United States have this problem. A study at Johns Hopkins Medical Center recently showed that two-thirds of patients there were intolerant of even a single glass of milk. It is well known that other cultures, especially in India and China, are broadly intolerant of milk, as are many American blacks. Because of genetic conditioning they do not have the enzymes necessary to assimilate milk. Inadvertent intake of milk makes them nauseous or constipated.

In addition, many people are allergic to milk, and the danger is that they attribute their problems to something else. Several researchers have shown that milk can also hinder the assimilation of nutrients in adults. Another interesting study showed that mothers who were breast feeding could relieve their babies' colic by eliminating milk from their own diets. And there are two other serious aspects of indiscriminate use of pasteurized milk:

1. Is milk irreplaceable by other nutrient sources, especially sources of calcium?
2. Is milk implicated in some way in heart disease?

A study by the Nutrition Biochemistry Laboratory of M.I.T. compared the health of children living in a middle-class suburb in Michigan with that of poor children in a Mexican village. Surprisingly, the Mexican children fared better overall, and without drinking milk they had higher calcium levels. The implication is not that milk isn't a good source of calcium, but that it isn't the *only* good source. The second question turns on the action of an enzyme, xanthine oxidase, which is transported in the blood by homogenized fat droplets and thereby allowed to damage the elasticity of arterial walls. Many researchers feel that this is the cause of atherosclerosis in teenagers, which was first observed to be quite common in autopsies of American soldiers during the Korean War. Without pasteurization, of course, there would be no homogenization, which is now almost universal. Research going back to 1933 has identified several other nutrient losses caused by pasteurization, notably vitamins A and D. Yet, in a textbook published recently by a professor at the University of California, the whole question is dismissed with a simple statement: "The prevention of disease and of the spread of disease by this means far outweigh any imagined dietary loss."

What should you do about milk? First, be aware that milk allergies and intolerances may be causing the problems you attribute to other allergies. Second, use it in moderation, a glass or two a day, supplemented by cheese and yogurt. Third, since it is a highly concentrated protein food, serve it alone rather than with other nutrient-rich foods. Fourth, keep other, less expensive and less concentrated liquids on hand for purposes of satisfying thirst—such as distilled water or, occasionally, diluted fruit juices. Fifth, don't imagine that by using skim milk you are overcoming any of the above problems; by removing the butterfat the processors have only taken a natural product one more step toward artificiality, and in fact research has shown that skim milk is harder to digest.

Textbooks such as the one referred to above form the basis of the training of dietitians; is it any wonder that processed food in its worst states makes up the diet of most hospitals? This particular text compounds misinformation with outright propaganda for the food industry. On a single page devoted to the question of food processing, we are told that the following statements are *myths*:

- Poor soil affects the nutritive content of the food grown on it.
- Organic manure as opposed to commercial chemicals makes a difference in the food's nutritional composition.
- Nutritive qualities of vitamins and minerals as they occur naturally in foods differ from those that are synthetically produced in a laboratory and added to food.
- Food processing destroys the nutritive value of food.

In reality, these statements are all *facts*! Staple crops such as rice and wheat are considerably depleted in nutrients as soil becomes depleted of minerals. Research has been conducted for several years on the differences between organic and chemical fertilizers and there is no question of whether there are differences, but only how great they are. On the third point, it is important to repeat here that nutrients always work synergistically, never in isolation, and that nothing we create in a laboratory and add to foods can take into account all the variables at work in the natural product. (It is this fact that explains best what we mean by a "whole" food. It is a food from which nothing has been removed, though, of course, some of its nutrients may have been diminished through natural attrition. One of the major tasks of a biochemist is to study the metabolic pathways of food. These pathways were developed over the eons of evolution when man was eating a diet of whole foods. It is therefore quite likely that nutrients will be assimilated more readily when taken as parts of whole foods.)

Finally, even food manufacturers agree that processing destroys nutrients in varying degrees. This is why, of course, they have "refortified" such foods as bread and milk.

The basic value you must seek in food purchasing is *maximum nutrient for the money*. The practical side of this is that foods that no one will eat, or eat much of, are of zero nutrient value. In the past generation or two, Americans have *junked* certain types of foods, either because "the kids won't eat liver" or because liver wasn't fashionable. There are styles in menu planning as there are in dress. Sweetbreads and squid, for example, two excellent, nutrient-rich foods, are now back in style—at least at the restaurant level. In general, as you are able to get more of the organ meats into your cooking (liver, heart, kidneys, etc.), you are feeding your family better, for less. But be practical: add these in ground form to hamburger, or use them in soups, as you use giblets in gravy. In general, use meat more sparingly—not because of its high animal fat content but because there are other, less expensive forms of protein: eggs, cheese, and combinations of vegetables. (Cheese is "predigested" in a sense, and so is less of a problem for one who is intolerant of milk.) Remember, soybeans pose a minor problem of possibly blocking the absorption of zinc and iron, but if other proteins are used with soy this obstacle is overcome. (The biochemistry behind the complementarity of proteins is too complex to go into here, but even dieticians would not quarrel with this statement.) In general, the foods with the lowest ratio of nutrient to cost are the heavily processed foods. There is no free lunch in convenience foods.

A second guiding principle for getting maximum nutrient value is to pattern your menus after ethnic meals. These "recipes" have stood the test of time. You will notice that grains are usually combined with vegetables to get a complete protein balance (tortilla and beans and rice and beans in Latin American cuisine, soybean and rice in Chinese dishes). Since most of the world is vegetarian, by choice or not, protein complementarity has been crucial to survival. (*Diet for a Small Planet* explains protein complementarity, and, along with *Laurel's Kitchen* that we've mentioned earlier, is one of the many good books that offer a complete approach to vegetarian food preparation and selection: See the Appendix I for these and other suggested readings.) The presence of garlic and other rich-tasting herbs in ethnic cooking likewise appears to be no accident. For years conventional thinking has considered the nutritional claims of garlic ("the poor man's penicillin") to be another old wives' tale. Old wives are being vindicated right and left these days: a recent study of two provinces in China has shown that garlic in the diet has preventive effects against gastric cancer. Nitrosamines, which are formed in the gut from nitrites and amines, are known carcinogens. It appears from the Chinese study that garlic significantly reduces nitrites in the stomach by inhibiting bacterial growth. (Incidentally, garlic can be used sparingly and still be effective nutritionally. Cooking with garlic is, of course, the traditional way to take it. Garlic tablets are available to preclude breath problems, but I believe in taking good foods "for better or for worse.")

Americans have *junked* the more difficult foods in favor of the bland, high-carbohydrate, high-sugar foods; the ethnic foods in favor of the fast foods; and more recently the "fatty" foods, such as eggs and butter, for the artificial foods, such as skim milk and margarine. It's time to go back to what has been time-tested in human evolution. And you can do it with simply a little extra resolve when you go shopping.

Poisons for a Small Planet

When Frances Moore Lappe opened the window on vegetarianism with her *Diet for a Small Planet,* she got women thinking again about food habits (men went their merry ways with 16-ounce steaks, blood rare). She has now taken up another cause, the spread of pesticides in our food. Her point is dramatic: we are poisoning ourselves by being unconcerned about the health of the rest of the world.

Certain pesticides, such as heptachlor, chlordane, and BHC, are prohibited in the United States, but can be manufactured here and sold abroad. Since warning instructions are sometimes not read in underdeveloped countries, pesticides in dangerous concentrations are used on foods that often find their way back to this country. It's a small world. So we have BHC in our morning coffee, and the DDT used on crops in El Salvador finds its way to Miami in beef carcasses. And at least 20 other pesticides for which the FDA has no reliable method of detection, all potential carcinogens, are being shipped overseas.

At least two other potent pesticides, lindane and carbon tetrachloride, are used in a number of products in the United States despite the fact that both are known carcinogens. Lindane is particularly prevalent in products for the home: flea collars, dog washes, floor wax, shelf paper. Although it is heavily used in lumbering and agriculture, residues seem to be at low levels *at the present time.* The problem is that numerous chemical fumes are already in the air in most homes (chlorine, paints, cleansers), and the combination of various fumes has an unpredictable outcome. You cannot singlehandedly change American policies about selling insecticides abroad, but you can avoid bringing poisons into your home now. And you can make your voice heard in a number of environmentalist organizations concerned about chemical pollution. The avoidance of pollution is as important in nourishing your family as is the avoidance of malnutrition.

The Last Word on Cholesterol

Most women take responsibility for their husbands' diet, and so the burden falls on them to decide what to do about cholesterol.

The first step is to separate what is known from what is speculated. Even the American Heart Association readily admits that the cholesterol-lowering diet they recommend is based on a good guess and is a matter of prudent behavior rather than hard fact. The evidence can be summed up succinctly: *some* people have trouble with cholesterol.

When one reviews the evidence for and against dietary cholesterol (as found primarily in animal fats, including butter, whole milk, liver, and eggs), one can only conclude that indeed "a little knowledge is a dangerous thing." It all began in the early 1950s with the now infamous Framingham study. This epidemiological review attempted to find a correlation between high serum cholesterol (as measured in the standard blood tests) and a higher incidence of heart disease (as evidenced by coronary thrombosis). Such a correlation did turn up, and other population analyses seemed to confirm the cholesterol-in-the-blood and heart attack connection. Since then, however, it has been shown convincingly that too many other factors in the study were uncontrolled. Among these were the health status in general of the participants and other dietary factors. As critics of the AHA position have repeatedly pointed out, other large-scale epidemiological observations show just the opposite of the Framingham study. These range from populations in India and China to Irish natives versus Irish-Americans, to Eastern European countries in industrialized and nonindustrialized regions. Moreover, such studies form only one link in the three-part chain supposedly connecting a high-fat diet with the risk of heart attack.

The chain under debate is this: (1) Does dietary intake of high-cholesterol foods raise blood cholesterol? (2) Does blood cholesterol increase the incidence of arteriosclerosis (the blockage of the arteries to the heart)? (3) Does arteriosclerosis cause heart attacks? Only the third link in this chain has been established beyond reasonable doubt. The Framingham study and others deal only with the second link. The AHA position leaps from the first link to the third.

The first link seems plausible, and its plausibility is the very reason why it has been so mindlessly accepted by the general public (and shamefully promoted by establishment medicine).

Whenever studies are cited to show that more eggs and steaks do not necessarily result in higher serum cholesterol levels, establishment watchdogs rail against the dairy industry or the meat producers for funding such studies. The facts are that the liver produces cholesterol for essential bodily functions whether you ingest high levels of cholesterol or not; that blood cholesterol levels go up dangerously on a high-fat diet *only for those people who already have dangerously high levels;* and that low levels of cholesterol are associated with a generally high mortality rate from all causes. In short, cholesterol is good, but some people, perhaps 10 percent of the population, have a lipid (fat) disorder in which high cholesterol intake is not properly regulated.

The Food and Nutrition Board of the National Research Council has taken the unequivocal position that normal Americans will not reduce the risk of heart attack by going on a low-fat, low-cholesterol diet. The AHA obviously feels that such a pronouncement will falsely encourage those with high cholesterol levels to go their merry way eating the fat on steaks. So by coercing the entire population into cutting out the fat they hope to catch that 10 percent who would be better off with less fat in the diet. This is like taking salt out of everyone's diet because for some people salt leads to hypertension, or like prescribing insulin for the entire population because there may be some diabetics out there who are not taking care of themselves.

The folly is compounded by the overzealousness of such organizations as the Center for Science in the Public Interest. Under the direction of biochemist Dr. Michael Jacobson, who has crusaded against chemical additives in foods, this Washington-based group publishes nutrition information that is widely disseminated. In the case of cholesterol, the CSPI has taken its lead from the AHA and the AMA rather than from the National Research Council, and in turn it is quoted as an authoritative source by newspaper and magazine columnists. The CSPI publishes a chart that purports to rate the nutritive value of popular foods. Understandably, this chart gives a minus rating to candy and ice cream. But it also rates butter, eggs, and whole milk low because of their cholesterol levels— three of the finest foods that have nourished us for eons. They should not become "junked foods" because of some late 20th-century dietary fad.

A sixty-six-year-old professor of family and community medicine, Margaret Flynn, is one of the growing corps of non-faddists who have taken to the media to fight the phobia over cholesterol. For more than a dozen years she has been keeping health records on some 600 of her fellow faculty and staff members at the University of Missouri. She has put them through a rigorous regimen of body-fat tests, periodic blood tests, and dietary experiments. Her conclusion is that in persons who have normal cholesterol levels to begin with, dietary changes—including three-month binges on all sorts of meat and eggs—have no effect on serum cholesterol.

Biochemist Dr. Richard Passwater has been the most outspoken critic of the second link in the supposed cholesterol–heart attack chain. He cites evidence to show that the "clogged pipe" model of arteriosclerosis is highly misleading. Arteries are more than rigid pipes; they are pulsing, living tissue. To become stopped up, they must first be damaged. Arteries have a layer of muscle between their inner and outer walls to increase the flow of oxygen by tightening the vessel. It is significant that veins, which do not have such a muscle, do not become blocked. The health of both the inner wall (intima) and the arterial muscle is critical to the free flow of blood. Cholesterol deposits found in clogged arteries are more likely the end products of cellular deterioration than the cause of the narrowing of the arteries. And this deterioration is caused by deficiencies in vitamins C and E as well as many other nutrients which build body tissue. Passwater concludes, "No matter how many eggs or pats of butter or glasses of milk you have dropped from your diet, you still have a 50 percent chance of dying prematurely from a heart attack. . . . If your diet is less than perfect and you don't exercise quite enough, then it's no longer a question of whether you will get heart disease, but how seriously and when."

The death rate from heart disease has dropped almost 25 percent since the early 1970s. The cholesterol witchhunters, blithely ignoring the fact that the egg scare began to take effect in the late 1950s, cite this fact as evidence that dietary fat reduction is accomplishing something. In reality, the general health consciousness of the American public—notably the popularization of vitamin C by Linus Pauling and the turn to aerobic

exercise—coincides with this reversal in heart attack statistics.
At a recent conference in San Francisco on nutrition, a group of
doctors was asked to show their opinions about the
cholesterol–heart disease connection with a show of hands. The
speaker asked, "Do you accept the Heart Association position?"
And when only a few scattered hands went up, he commented,
"This is the reaction I've been getting lately."

Perhaps the last word on the cholesterol issue has come
from a year-long test of the Pritikin low-fat diet and the AHA
limited-fat diet (currently recommended: 30 percent or less
fat). In this Canadian study of patients with the beginnings of
vascular disease, *neither* diet lowered blood cholesterol. Dr.
Gordon D. Brown, clinical professor of medicine at the University
of Alberta, was asked what diet he would recommend as a
result of his study. "I'd recommend exercise," he answered.

Diet as a Teaching Aid

The cholesterol controversy should teach homemakers a basic
rule: don't give in to any food fad. The reason why children are
undernourished and their fathers are prey to heart disease is
that those who shop and prepare food have been victimized by
the center aisles, the packaged food locations, of the grocery
store. And children *are* undernourished in this country, despite
the assurances of the food industry. One study after another
has turned up vitamin and mineral deficiencies in adolescents.
In the most recent, teenagers from a blue-collar neighborhood
in New York City were carefully monitored and tested for eating
habits and levels of the vital B vitamin riboflavin. This is one of
the vitamins, you remember, that has been put back in "enriched" bread. Deficiency states were noted in a significant percentage of the children. An interesting finding was that many of
them drank less than one cup of milk a *week*—quite a measure
of malnutrition in this country—and those were the ones who
were seriously depleted of riboflavin (which is available in fairly
good quantities in milk).

A corollary of not giving in to fads is not to go to extremes.
You will recall the discussion of the dangers of high intake of
milk. This hardly implies that giving up milk, except in the case

of intolerance or an allergy, is a good idea. When one begins to shop along the walls of the supermarket, where whole foods usually are, instead of in the aisles, the diet necessarily becomes more varied. It is difficult to eat any one food—if it's a whole food and not a processed food—to excess.

Mothers should take their children shopping with them, to show them why they choose certain foods. When one goes on a diet, one should look for general principles rather than recipes. Any diet that fails to teach you something is not worthy of the name. Mothers should also teach their children the dangers of certain foods—even whole foods. For example, potatoes that are green can be poisonous to one degree or another even after being cooked; margarines and vegetable oils, which supposedly save you from the dangers of butter, can become high in *trans* fats as they are heated in meal preparation. (See Chapter 12 for more on this issue.) And there is a psychological truth here that every woman should know as a matter of routine: the more you try to teach, the more you learn.

9

New Hope in Coping with Alcohol

A documentary film on women, drugs, and alcohol, "The Last to Know," recently focused attention on a problem that is symptomatic of society's approach to the health concerns of women. We deny that anything's wrong. Just as premenstrual syndrome has been ignored until recent years, the specter of the woman alcoholic has been too much for our sensibilities to handle. Fortunately, a few prominent women have come forward to talk about their alcoholism. But it will be many years before the millions of "invisible" alcoholics who also happen to be female receive the same sympathetic treatment and concern that the typical heavy-drinking businessman now enjoys. Yes, millions: as this excellent film makes clear, of the estimated 10 million alcoholics in the United States today, nearly *half* are women.

Given the fact that men have traditionally been exposed to many more opportunities to drink, it seems preposterous that nearly half the alcoholics are women. Is this a recent phenomenon, similar to smoking and lung cancer in women? To some extent, yes; it is now equally acceptable for women to drink, and perhaps more feasible for those who feel trapped in a home with an abundant liquor cabinet. Yet I doubt that this is the only reason, or even that the phenomenon is all that recent. Government figures show that the per capita consumption of alcohol, measured in proof rather than liquid volume, "did not change significantly during the years 1971 to 1976." A slight increase has begun to be noticeable since then, but nothing to indicate a large number of women entering the drinking scene. The same source shows "little overall increase" in mortality rates from alcoholism (about 2 per 100,000) nor in alcoholic psychosis rates (about 1 per 100,000) in the 25-year period from 1950 to 1975. Likewise, studies of teenagers of both sexes in recent years have not turned up the expected increase in the regularity or quantity of alcoholic consumption by young people—although this other "invisible" problem has recently received much publicity. Rather, I think that women have always suffered more than the medical fraternity would admit, even though women perhaps do not drink as heavily as men. The reasons lie in the particular health needs of women and, conversely, in their victimization by overprescribed drugs.

Women are given many more prescription drugs than men. They are more susceptible, as we have seen, to common depression and anxiety. In addition, their more active hormonal state and the cycle of their reproductive system place heavy demands on nutrients. All of these factors are in some way interrelated—and nutrient-depletion in them all has this to do with alcoholism: it is the common precursor of the "disease." Thus, the nutrient therapies that are effective in preventing the problems associated with drugs, with psychiatric disorders, or with the menstrual cycle also prevent or cope with the onset of alcoholic addiction and alcoholic deterioration of vital organs of the body.

It is interesting to note, in this often confusing disease state and contrary to the usual prescriptions for treatment, that the most common precursor of alcoholism is simply heavy drinking. It is usually assumed that the two are the same, or that heavy drinking simply is part of a continuum with alcoholism. But what heavy drinking actually does is so debilitate the nutritional condition of the drinker that he or she becomes defenseless against a whole array of illnesses that we lump together as alcoholism. Some people do not need to drink very much at all to become alcoholic; this is especially true of women who already suffer from the other precursor states mentioned above.

It can also be said, of course, that alcoholism is more than the depletion of B vitamins, the destruction of brain cells, or damage to the liver. It is also uniquely addictive. In this sense, it is like an allergy, or what might be called a biochemical addiction. But it is also psychologically addictive. The perspective of nutrient therapy has given us quite a bit of insight into the mechanisms of alcoholism, so that now we can answer the age-old questions about to what degree it is a disease, a failure of will, an allergy, a genetic trait, or simply an example of bad eating habits. As we have paid closer attention to women's alcoholism we have begun to see how the complex parts of the puzzle fit together.

Alcohol—Phantom Nutrient and Flagrant Poison

Because alcohol provides calories without nutrient values, it is very much like sugar and refined white flour. Thus, though it may give a sense of immediate energy, it not only fails to provide nutrients for cell growth but also interferes with the absorption of vitamins and amino acids and places greater burdens on the hormonal system. The heavy drinker can't "listen to her body" because her energy needs seem fulfilled. At the same time, alcohol actively damages various organs, such the pancreas and the liver, and can permanently disrupt the nervous system. The most publicized malady—cirrhosis of the liver—affects at most only a third of all chronic alcoholics, and can be caused by many things other than drinking. Yet its mechanism is clear-cut: acetylaldehyde, one of the products of ethanol, is directly toxic to the liver. Alcohol not only causes fat to be deposited in the liver by stimulating various hormones, but restricts the liver's ability to carry off fat by inhibiting the liver's functions, including protein production. The organ becomes infiltrated with fat, and as they become inflamed, liver cells die. This hepatitis condition leads to the scar formation that gives cirrhosis its name. A physician can diagnose a swollen or fatty liver in a physical examination, but any heavy drinker (more than a pint of 80-proof liquor or its equivalent a day) will have such symptoms as abdominal distress, bleeding (as evidenced in tarry, black stools), unsteadiness, frequent mental lapses, and inability to concentrate.

It is well understood that alcohol offers its social benefits by being rapidly absorbed into the bloodstream and entering the brain. Within five to twenty minutes after taking a single drink, blood levels of alcohol are measurable. What is not so widely known is that the effect of alcohol on the brain is to *depress the central nervous system*. A social drinker becomes more excitable after a few drinks not because she is stimulated but because her inhibitions are depressed. Fast repartee results from the relaxation of tension rather than from the excitation of the mental network. And the depression of the central nervous system is akin to depression in general, a slowing down of all the bodily functions. Thus it is that alcoholics have 55 times the suicide rate of non-alcoholics. The alcohol that reaches the brain—and it reaches the brain in great quantities because the brain requires so much blood—can paralyze the cells that serve for short-term memory and accelerate their destruction. These and other cells throughout the body require large amounts of folic acid for repair—a nutrient that is seldom supplied in sufficient quantities even in vitamin-mineral supplements.

This is the bad news. The not-so-bad news is that alcohol is better in some forms than in others, and that in moderate amounts can have positive health benefits. The distilled form of alcoholic drinks—"hard liquor" typically 80 or 86 proof—not only has no nutrient value but also has impurities that compound the effects of alcohol. Beer and wine, which achieve their alcoholic level through natural fermentation, have sufficient food value to require some digestion by the body. Wine, for example, has trace minerals and bioflavonoids (especially if nonpasteurized), while beer has the residue of brewer's yeast, chiefly the minerals silicon and chromium. Beer also has the favorable property of being a sort of purified water that is rapidly absorbed into the tissues, precisely because of its alcoholic content. The relaxant effects of these beverages are generally appreciated; one French oenophile has gone so far as to suggest certain vintages for certain maladies. Yet it cannot be denied that wine stimulates the appetite and aids the digestion (aperitif and digestif), for those who need it, especially the elderly. The most recent scientific addition to this treasure trove of folk wisdom is that a few drinks a day, up to 1½ ounces of pure alcohol, appears to improve one's longevity statistically vis-à-vis teetotalers. (A beer contains about ½ ounce of alcohol, as does a glass of wine or a mixed drink. Remember, 80 proof means 40 percent alcohol.) The Johns Hopkins study that provided this news did not, unfortunately, assay the nutritional difference between alcohol in the form of beer or wine and in the form of hard liquor. Nor did it attempt to assay the effect on longevity of other characteristics of nondrinkers.

The paradox of simultaneous euphoria and depression is only the first of many confusing aspects of drinking. There are several tests one can take to measure one's chances of becoming an alcoholic—for example, the questionnaires used by Alcoholics Anonymous about when, why, and in what emotional states you take a drink. There are psychological and chemical forms of treatment—popularly, Alcoholics Anonymous and Antabuse. Surprisingly, the treatment that has seemed most obvious as the basis for other modalities is only now seeing widespread acceptance. This is nutrient therapy, and it has taken three apparently unrelated forms: the allergy hypothesis of Dr. Theron G. Randolph; the prostaglandin studies of Dr. David F. Horrobin; and the broad nutritional program of Dr. Roger J. Williams. What is fascinating about all three approaches is their particular application to women.

Thirty Years of Neglect

In the early 1950s Dr. Williams published his first reports on the nutritional approach to treating alcoholism. He was then able to assist Dr. Frederick Stare at Harvard in setting up a controlled experiment of the effects of vitamin supplements on alcoholics. Dr. Stare is a well-known professor with strong conservative views in this field; it was therefore promising when the *Journal of the American Medical Association* reported favorably on this work in 1954:

> There is evidence that not all the patients took the medication prescribed, and this factor inevitably operates to diminish the apparent effectiveness of the treatment. . . . Some persons

are benefited by vitamin therapy. The results are sufficiently favorable to warrant additional research on the effects of nutritional supplements in the treatment of alcoholism and on the studies of metabolism of alcohol.

Dr. Williams described the failure of medical research to follow up on this lead as "pathetic." As of this writing, there has still been no subsequent testing of the vitamin-therapy hypothesis, yet nowadays we know much more about how such research might proceed.

We know, for example, that the handful of vitamins used in the 1954 study was woefully inadequate and did not even raise the question of mineral supplementation. There is no doubt today that zinc and magnesium play critical roles in the treatment of alcoholics. Most importantly, this early effort was flawed by a lack of understanding of the biochemical individuality of each human being. Whereas the ranges of the RDAs seem to imply that individuals differ only by 50 to 100 percent, in the studies done by Williams it has been shown that one person may require *six or seven times* the amounts of a particular vitamin or mineral needed by another. It is not at all surprising, therefore, that the Harvard study was inconclusive. What is surprising is that the anti-vitamin establishment has used this study to support their skepticism!

As I have mentioned several times before, there is a greater range of biochemical variation among women than among men. This fact suggests that women might be more susceptible to the chain of events leading to alcoholism: persistent drinking, nutrient deficiency, and metabolic breakdown. It is a commonplace of observation that some people are able to drink regularly without any obvious problems, while others cannot afford to take that first one. Dr. Williams and his researchers have concentrated their efforts on identifying the metabolic differences in individuals that can account for this extreme variation. The results make an obvious case for the biochemical origin of alcoholism and hence for the nutritional approach to prevention and cure.

As far back as 1949 Dr. Williams and his coworkers were able to show that laboratory animals could be induced to choose alcohol freely if certain vitamins were eliminated from their diets. One by one, vitamins A, B_1, B_2, B_6, and pantothenic acid were removed and then restored to their feed, and as each vitamin was removed the animals "took to drink" and as each vitamin was restored they went back to abstinence. By careful urinary examinations the researchers were able to identify remarkable variations in the metabolism of these animals. It was therefore clear that these commonly available vitamins were only the gross causative factors in susceptibility to alcohol. Similar urinary patterns in children were then studied, and it was found that significant correlations existed between specific metabolic patterns and behavior problems. Other research began to converge on the hypothesis that the brain—and hence the substances that critically affect the brain—are the major signals of biochemical individuality. Ethnic groups differed widely in their ability, en masse, to handle alcohol. Amino acid patterns in the blood later were available for exacting measurement with the advent of chromatography—and these too showed wide-ranging variations, this time from individual to individual. Dr. Mary K. Roach showed that the brain's ability to handle glucose, its prime fuel, is adversely affected by alcohol, and much more adversely in some individuals than in others. Finally, Dr. Eleanor Storrs was able to show that even in identical twins the hormone levels and amino acid levels could differ by factors of two or more in the mammalian brain. This latter study, incidentally, shows how deep biochemical individuality runs and how radically we must revise our conception of inherited traits. The nub of Dr. Williams's argument from these studies can be summarized as follows:

1. The inability to handle alcohol is related to brain function.
2. Great individual differences exist from one person to the next in the brain functions of utilizing certain vitamins, glucose, and amino acids, among other things
3. Animal experiments and a limited number of human observations connect these functions with the presence or absence of alcohol.

There is no longer any doubt that alcohol depletes the same vitamins which, when they are deficient, tend to *induce* the ingestion of alcohol. This is a curious effect, and it does not have any obvious parallel in medicine or nutrition. If you have low blood sugar, you will tend to want to eat simple carbohydrates; but eating simple carbohydrates further reduces your blood sugar level by overstimulating the insulin reaction of the pancreas. Whereas if you are anemic it is because of a deficiency of iron; but the symptoms of anemia do not cause an iron deficiency. The allergic mechanism, as we will see, comes closer to the alcohol-vitamin interconnection. But it is not clear that the latter can be understood as an allergy. What we do know from Dr. Williams's research, covering a lifetime of clinical as well as laboratory experience, is that several general nutritional rules must be at the core of any meaningful attack on alcoholism. He posits seven rules, which are listed on page 136. One of the seven requires a brief introduction.

A colleague of Dr. Williams, Professor William Shive, discovered some years ago that the poisoning effect of alcohol does not work against bacterial cells when certain foods are added to the reaction. Alcohol in sufficient quantities stops bacteria from multiplying. But when extracts of liver, cabbage, and certain other foods were added to the bacterial culture, bacteria were able to grow readily. He was able to isolate the substance that was common to these foods—the amino acid glutamine. Further experiments showed that glutamine, in contrast to all the 21 other amino acids, inhibits laboratory animals from drinking alcohol. The other amino acids and all other nutrients tested have not yet shown this effect. Further trials with alcoholics since 1958 have confirmed the animal studies, and Dr. Williams and his colleagues have received numerous testimonials from alcoholics who have been helped with daily doses of glutamic acid, in the form of a small, inexpensive tablet. But why should this single substance have such results? Biochemist Dr. Richard Passwater explains:

> Glutamic acid is not made into brain chemicals called neurotransmitters, as are some amino acids, nor is glutamic acid incorporated into protein structure in the brain. Glutamic acid has two major functions. The unique surprise is that glutamic acid serves primarily as a fuel for the brain, a feat which only one other compound, glucose (blood sugar), can perform. The second major function of glutamic acid is . . . to pick up excess ammonia.

Since excess ammonia can cause brain damage, it is reasonable to suppose that this protective function of glutamic acid (or L-glutamate) is what we see when alcoholics report better functioning after regular doses of the substance. On the other hand, the fact that glutamic acid provides brain fuel may explain why alcoholics turn away from liquor after taking it: they no longer need the "instant glucose" that alcohol provides. In short, glutamic acid gives us a model to explain that "curious effect" I mentioned above concerning nutrients in general vis-à-vis alcohol. Nutrients in general, and L-glutamate in particular, have more than one function in the brain, and are affected by more than one antagonist. Thus the medical literature contains reports of benefits of glutamic acid with mentally deficient children, in appetite control, in ulcers, in petit mal epilepsy, in mental disorders of various kinds, and in impotence.

The first and basic rule that Dr. Williams lays down in his most recent book, *The Prevention of Alcoholism Through Nutrition*, is to realize that you are unique biochemically. One or more of the remaining six rules may work for you, but not for others. Second, you may find that you do not have a glutamic acid deficiency—but give this nutrient a try. Third, you may not need vitamin and mineral supplements—but this is often a helpful preventive measure. Fourth, concentrate on high-quality foods, and fifth, avoid low-quality foods, and you may not have any deficiencies that would call for a nutritional supplement. Sixth, exercise to promote internal nutrition. Seventh, cultivate moderation and inner peace as a way of life.

Even after 30 years or more of neglect of Dr. Williams's broad program by institutional medicine, he is far from angry or frustrated. In *The Prevention of Alcoholism Through Nutrition*, he acknowledges all the reasons why physicians have treated alcoholism as something alien to scientific medical practice. He concludes: "The deficiencies of the medical profession with respect to alcoholism are the result of neither consistent stupidity nor a villainous plot."

The Allergy Model of Alcoholism

Dr. Theron G. Randolph is known throughout the world as a pioneer in allergy studies. Yet, like Dr. Williams, he finds that a host of factors in our society and educational system have blinded the medical profession to this approach to alcoholism. In a recent interview he said almost in desperation, "Despite the fact that the connection between alcoholism and food allergy has been confirmed by Dr. Richard Macarness in England, by Dr. Marshall Mandell in Connecticut, and several others, no person active in the teaching or handling of alcoholism has displayed the slightest interest in this point of view."

Women are in a far better position to appreciate food allergies than are men. Not only do they suffer from them more often, as a result of their greater biochemical individuality, but they are exposed to foods in a greater variety of forms in the home. Furthermore, mothers are exposed to the allergies of their children and in general have been the victims of closed environments. Anyone who spends most of the day in the same room or set of rooms is more likely to develop a food addiction than one who has a change of air, liquids, and eating situations from day to day. Dr. Randolph has shown conclusively that allergic reactions to certain foods, notably corn, can be a hidden but quite prominent cause of what we think of as alcoholism. It is easy to see how this kind of "drinking problem" can account for many cases of alcoholism that don't seem to have any relation to the heavy drinking that many men do.

Corn is a major ingredient in some bourbons, and various other grains are used in the manufacture of everything from beer to rye. Dr. Randolph has discovered, however, that minute amounts of grains are used in other ways in the liquor industry. Corn syrup is used to provide the right color for apple and grape brandies; corn is imported by Scotland to give their whiskies the bourbonized flavor that Americans prefer. But even if the offending allergen is not present in the liquor, alcohol has the ability to transport any food in the stomach to the bloodstream about three times faster than it would otherwise be so absorbed. This rapid absorption of an allergic food, either in the liquor itself or riding along with the alcohol, can produce the specific concentration of the allergen needed to cause a reaction. People who become quite intoxicated on a drink or two may be the victims of their biochemical individuality, as Dr. Williams proposes; but they may also be victims of innate or acquired allergies. The woman who becomes red in the face or feels a sharp tingle under her jaw after the first drink cannot be brushed aside as just an inexperienced drinker. If a few more drinks remove those sensations, she could be experiencing what is known as the classic "masked food allergy."

Dr. Herbert Rinkel first identified this phenomenon. In most allergies, he explained, the foreign body, the antigen (anti-gene), precipitates the production of antibodies by the immune system. (The histamine that is released when invading bodies attack signals T-cells in the thymus gland to counterattack, either with protein molecules or antibodies.) Not only do the T-cells "remember" this event, but they also magnify the immune response under heavy stimulation by activating other protective cells, the B-lymphocytes. Thus one can get a violent reaction to shellfish or penicillin, or in more common cases to poison oak or ivy. The immediate inflammation is so obvious that the victim avoids the food or foreign substance then and there and thereafter. But, Rinkel noticed, in less pronounced allergic reactions the victim learns to cover up the pain (inflammation, headache, sneezing) by ingesting *more* of the offending substance to trigger more of a response. In the case of alcohol, withdrawal symptoms and sometimes a hangover are such pains, and "the hair of the dog" is the antidote. Thus the victim masks the cause of the allergy by wallowing in the cause. Dr. Randolph rightly points out that in this instance it is more to the point to call the allergy an addiction.

Many of Dr. Randolph's patients drank bourbon only to mask the effects of the corn in the bourbon. He notes that many reformed alcoholics develop a craving for candy, to get the corn syrup in the candy. And, of course, the masking effect can occur without reference to alcohol. The most common example is a wheat allergy. The patient insists, "But doctor, I *love* bread. How can I be allergic to it?" Whenever I hear a patient say that she just can't handle alcohol, but frequently goes overboard, I suspect an allergy to something, however inconspicuous, in what she drinks or in what she adds to her drinks.

Is alcoholism *explained* by allergies? Are all addictions a form of allergy? Not at all. Alcohol indulgence is caused by a variety of factors, and so is treatable by one or several approaches. There is no question that the psychological pressures that women face as "trapped" housewives, or as thwarted professionals, or as rejected mothers can be the catalysts that drive them to drink. Can the unusually severe incidence of alcoholism in the Scandinavian countries and the Soviet Union be explained by a potato allergy, or are the stresses of their various social systems to blame?

A recent case of mine illustrates how many factors may be interwoven in a drinking problem. Jeanine is a career woman who moved to San Francisco from New York in a promotion in her advertising agency. She seemed to have everything going for her, including health and good looks. But she came to me on the recommendation of a friend because of problems that were visible only to her. She did a considerable amount of drinking in connection with entertaining clients. This, she thought, brought on the sleepiness in the afternoon and the midmorning chronic fatigue. Coffee in the morning gave her a pick-me-up, and a few glasses of white wine at lunch let her down. This cycle was continued with other caffeine drinks in the late afternoon (cola or tea) and she relaxed in the evening with more wine. She was taking a drugstore-type vitamin supplement, but smoked almost a pack of cigarettes a day. Her exercise consisted of tennis and occasional racketball. Little by little, she felt herself falling apart.

The seriousness of her condition became apparent during her glucose tolerance test, in which she had blurred vision and nearly fainted. And her history showed considerable stress both at work and in her personal life: marital problems caused by her moving, competition with men in the agency, worry about her dependence on alcohol. And little things began to add up: a high pulse rate of 84, barely 1,200 calories daily in her diet (as determined by computer analysis), and frequent headaches. It is a tribute to her self-awareness that she would come to a doctor with such vague symptoms. When she saw that she had a problem with low blood sugar, her trip was justified.

On the controlled carbohydrate diet she showed immediate improvement, including a definite desire to limit her drinking. The mega-nutrition vitamin and mineral program I prescribed, together with more aerobic exercise, gradually dissipated her desire to smoke. After a month and a half, she said something to me that hits right at the heart of typical cases like hers: "When you feel better you like yourself better."

There is also no doubt that by lowering her carbohydrate intake and producing ketones she was providing a reserve source of fuel for her brain! As we have seen, glucose and glutamine are the only normal fuel for the brain; but ketones are the reserve fuel tank that nature has prepared for us in such situations as starvation. I strongly suspect that she had difficulty utilizing glucose, and that ketones came to the rescue. Her headaches gone, her blood sugar stabilized, she said, "I have more energy in my life than ever. I'm handling things better." She no longer needed something like alcohol to hang on to: "the bottle" had been preferable to what she was experiencing in her daily life.

For many people, alcohol is simply the best deal they have found in life's little stresses. When they find something better, they no longer drink.

The New Hope of Prostaglandins

Dr. David F. Horrobin of Montreal is a leading researcher in the relatively new and exciting field of prostaglandins. Only a few years ago it would have seemed far-fetched to make the statement, "Prostaglandins (PGs) are very short-lived substances which seem to regulate the function of every cell in the body." Yet this is precisely how Dr. Horrobin began the lead story in Sweden's prestigious journal of metabolic medicine. (It is interesting to note that most of Europe is more advanced than the United States in accepting orthomolecular medicine. In Germany, the largest medical society is oriented to nutritional practice.)

As we mentioned in Chapter 3, prostaglandins act as messengers of pain, and are blocked by aspirin. But, as Dr. Horrobin points out, PGs have all sorts of effects—on the immune system, on blood pressure, on insulin, on platelets, on calcium deposits, on inflammation. This is because PGs are of three types, and there are many subgroups among these types. One of the type-one PGs, PGE1, has two remarkable benefits (among others): the relief of the symptoms of premenstrual syndrome, and the prevention of the withdrawal syndrome in alcoholism!

Much of the literature on PGE1 is scientifically complex, but the benefits of increased PGE1 production are clear-cut. Even a brief and simplified account of how PGE1 is produced shows the interrelationship of nutrients in the body. Essential fatty acids (EFAs) in food are the starting point. EFAs are found in abundance in vegetable oils, dairy products, and organ meats. A common EFA, cis-linoleic acid, is converted to an acid, GLA, by a key enzyme, D6D, and in turn converted to the acid DGLA. Zinc, vitamin B_6, and magnesium are all needed in this process, and now vitamin C is required to convert DGLA to PGE1. Various factors can also inhibit this metabolic pathway, among them *trans* fats (produced when fats are heated), a high blood glucose level, and chronic drinking. Trans fatty acids are a sort of "mixed up" EFA that result from heat and catalytic processing, especially in bakery products, margarines, and cooked vegetable oils. Trans fats not only are metabolically useless in this pathway, but undermine it. So in our "diet of commerce" we run the risk of running short of the very useful prostaglandin, PGE1. In controlled studies, PGE1 offered either dramatic or substantial relief in almost 90 percent of cases of premenstrual tension. Earlier in this chapter I mentioned the "curious effect" of alcohol depleting the very vitamins which, when present, discourage drinking. In this case a similarly curious effect occurs: alcohol depletes PGE1, and when PGE1 is stimulated by some other means it diminishes the bad effects of alcohol— even hangovers!

It is, in fact, critical to have some other means of increasing PGE1 production when various antagonists, including the lack of crucial vitamins and minerals, constantly threaten its metabolic pathway. The vulnerable link in the pathway is D6D. Dr. Horrobin and others have found that this link can be bypassed to provide GLA directly. Thus far, only two foods have been discovered to do this: mother's milk and evening primrose oil.

When I explained this to a friend, she was not surprised at all that mother's milk would contain this vital ingredient. But evening primrose oil? "You're putting me on!" she said. Yet it's true. Two commercial versions of this natural food are now on the market, Efamol and Preglandin. Research is now under way at several sites to expand on the studies and leads we now have. It seems clear to me that alcoholism in women may be the major focus of this research in terms of immediate benefits, for the factors behind premenstrual syndrome are not unrelated to the psychological and biochemical reasons why women drink to excess.

Dr. Horrobin's work in this field is a model of what nutrient therapy has to offer where conventional medicine is helpless. In his own words,

Investigation of sophisticated nutritional techniques for manipulating the endogenous biochemical pathways in the body is only just beginning. It seems likely to be a technique for maintaining health which has an excellent future.

10

Eat Right for Easy Exercise

Ten years ago, there was only one thing you could say about exercise: it burned up calories and perhaps firmed your muscles. You were told that it would take a half hour of jogging or an hour of walking to burn off the effects of one ice cream sundae. Even an ice cream cone cost you a half hour of brisk walking. It was obviously a poor way to overcome a weight problem. But then the aerobics movement began to take hold, and researchers began to look more deeply into the effects of exercise. What we now know is rather startling: sustained exercise does at least three helpful things:

1. It changes the way you make use of nutrients.
2. It changes the way your body burns its stores of energy.
3. It changes the way you eat, drink, and smoke.

It remains true, of course, that exercise burns, or, better said, accounts for, calories. Calories are so much on everyone's mind that this measure of energy is often thought of as some sort of food value—like proteins, fats, or carbohydrates. As we will see, calories are only a *measure,* and often a deceptive measure, of the energy value of food and the energy expenditure of human activity. As a rough estimate, it takes 3,500 calories of energy or of decreased food intake to lose a pound of weight. Calories *do* count, but they are far from the ironclad guide we once thought.

Women have every reason to be miffed at the way calorie-counting has dominated their idea of exercise. Already shunted away from vigorous athletics ("you'll develop muscles, look masculine, disrupt your internal organs," the old books used to say), they have been sold on exercise mainly to develop their busts, their legs, or their posture. Even the best of the TV fitness promoters, such as Jack LaLanne, talked mainly about "firming" and "getting ready for that summer swimsuit." In the mid-70s, we must remind ourselves, a woman who dared jump into the Boston Marathon was forcibly removed.

Times have changed, yet women account for only one of twenty runners who sign up for popular long-distance runs. They are more evident on the tennis court than on bicycles. They are still the most obvious victims of weight-loss clinics and "physician-supervised" crash diet schemes. Ironically, they have the most to gain from the simplest form of exercise program—aerobics—and they have the greatest access to a method of eating for fitness—the Listen to Your Body diet.

Women, Body Fat, and Aerobics

It is not uncommon for a woman to be measured at 30 percent body fat. Most men who are in reasonably good shape have 20 percent or less. Long-distance runners often are under 10 percent. One's exercise level alone doesn't account for this difference: in the biological scheme of things women's bodies have been outfitted with fatty tissues necessary for sustaining a pregnancy. And one's body type and climatic environment also predispose one for more or less fat. Yet body fat is still a better measure of essential fitness than weight. Other than providing a reserve store of energy, fat is a noncontributing part of one's body: it takes more energy to go through the day's chores carrying this extra load.

The only meaningful measurement of body fat, given the genetic factors that predispose women in general and some women in particular to higher levels, is a "before and after" test. At the beginning of your exercise program, if you have any doubts about your health at all, you should arrange for a treadmill or stress test and a body fat test. The stress test is a method of monitoring your vital signs while your exercise level—running on a treadmill—is systematically increased. You can thus safely determine your maximum heart rate, and thereafter you should limit aerobic exercise to a level of about three-quarters of that rate. Primarily, however, this test will uncover any preexisting heart conditions that would preclude taking up vigorous exercise. A key measure of your capacity for exercise is how rapidly your pulse returns to normal after a vigorous workout; this is a measure of the efficiency of your cardiovascular system. A complete stress test would also include a measurement of your oxygen uptake and lung capacity, both of which can be improved somewhat with extended exercise. Finally, the body fat measurement, done either by a skin-pinch test or by being weighed while totally immersed in a water tank, sets a benchmark against which you can chart your progress in improving your body composition.

I have mentioned the stress test almost peripherally because I think it's easy to lose sight of the main purpose of aerobic exercise in a plethora of numbers. Most women who are in normal good health will be able to tell quite readily what a comfortable and safe level of exercise is for them. It's usually about twice the normal pulse rate for maximum effect on the cardiovascular system: this is the level at which one can speak of the "training effect." And that level will approximate three-quarters of the maximum pulse rate you achieve on a treadmill. The point is to "listen." Listen for signs of stress, such as difficulty in breathing, redness in the face, soreness in the joints. Bill Bowerman, the famed Oregon track coach who was one of the prime movers in getting America jogging, has laid down two excellent rules that should be enough for anyone who finds it inconvenient or expensive to have a treadmill test:

1. Train, don't strain.
2. Jog or run at a speed at which you can still carry on a conversation.

The skin-fold thickness test for body fat can be done by a physician with a high degree of precision, but a woman can roughly gauge her own fitness by observing her "bulges" in the four areas the doctor examines. The easiest place to examine is the upper arm. Pinch the skin at the midpoint of the outside of the arm and at the front and back of the arm muscles (biceps and triceps). If you are relatively low in body fat, you will be able to grasp only a bit of skin fold between your thumb and forefinger in these three places. The thicker the fold, the more body fat. A physician would also check the skin above the pelvis and just below the shoulder blade. Again, the exactness of the measurement isn't the point; but whether you have a penchant for tests and measurements or not, you should try to become conscious of your body and how it can improve with exercise.

I mentioned above that women have the most to gain from and the easiest access to aerobic exercise, and perhaps now this is self-evident. They generally have freer access to foods of their choice. Most important, they have more body fat to lose, and they have in aerobics a form of exercise that is tailored to their lifestyle. Aerobic exercise can take the form of walking, alternate walking and jogging, running, cycling, swimming, cross-country skiing, or—and this is my point—*any* activity that raises the pulse rate to about twice normal for an extended period of time. The next question, then, is, How long is "extended"?

Various researchers have shown that the body has certain plateaus at which training effects are maximized. At 30 minutes, the benefits to the cardiovascular system are about ideal. At 10 minutes, these benefits are about half as much as at 30 minutes. Extending aerobic exercise to an hour adds perhaps only 20 percent to the benefits of 30 minutes. On the other hand, the cyclist or runner who is able to maintain her high pulse rate for two hours reaches another plateau—at which body fat becomes an important fuel, since carbohydrates are usually exhausted by then. In fact, the ability of long-distance runners to metabolize fat as fuel is what separates competitive marathoners from everyday joggers. Putting together all these figures about the plateaus that occur at 30 minutes and at two hours, we can see the reason why alternating short with long periods of exercise seems to be most beneficial. Finally, it should be pointed out that muscular fitness is achieved only by the breaking down and building up of cells (exercise physiologists have a device that enables you actually to hear the cells "popping" as you contract a muscle). When muscle cells have not had a chance to build back up completely, further exercise is partially wasted. An ideal strategy for aerobic exercise would accordingly include these general rules:

1. For most people, exercising every other day or three times weekly is adequate and perhaps better than a daily routine, as long as the exercise is at least 30 minutes. Muscles can then rebuild most effectively.
2. Alternating 30-minute periods of aerobic work with two-hour periods maximizes a woman's ability to burn body fat.
3. Combining various forms of aerobic activity can help a woman achieve these extended periods of exercise without risk of injuries.

The exponents of each method of aerobic exercise seldom consider the last point. The key element in aerobics is time, not distance or speed. It has been calculated that regardless of the speed of running, the caloric output is about 0.8 calories per pound, per mile. For competitive runners, workouts at a racing speed do improve one's performance; but we're concerned here with cardiovascular fitness. Caloric output is related directly to the flow of blood to muscles and their surrounding fat. This blood flow increases by about two-thirds in any sort of prolonged exercise, and brings with it certain hormones, such as adrenaline, and enzymes which break down fatty deposits. A woman can jog for ten minutes, lie down and do situps for a few minutes, do some gardening at a brisk pace for another ten minutes, and easily put together her 30 minutes of aerobics for the day. If she has a home or apartment to take care of, or any of the common drudgeries of raising a family, with a little planning she can work these chores into a program of jogging or swimming to achieve an occasional two-hour period of aerobics. The fat-burning process goes on regardless of the type of exercise, as long as it is aerobic and prolonged.

Women realize that, unlike men, they tend to gain weight in sexually significant parts of their bodies. Fat shows up first in a woman's breasts, hips, and buttocks. Fortunately, it is also true that women do not have the types of hormones that stimulate the growth of muscle mass, and their cells have fewer nuclei than those of males. This is why women can exercise and increase their strength without increasing muscle mass appreciably. Aerobic exercise is therefore psychologically more acceptable to women because it can accomplish the most for their good looks without the hazards of injury or strain that are associated with competitive sports or weight training.

The Added Bonuses of Aerobic Exercise

There is scarcely a book or magazine article on diet and exercise that does not promise rewards for "just a few minutes a day." This is nonsense; there is no magic that can shorten the time you must spend on aerobic workouts! On the other hand, there do seem to be some unexpected bonuses in aerobics other than what we have just seen in cardiovascular fitness and fat metabolism. But first consider the promises of those who are not taken with aerobics.

Walking has always been one of the safest and easiest forms of exercise. Unfortunately, it's not truly aerobic in the sense that it doesn't usually get the pulse up to 140 or more. The advocates of walking over jogging breeze past this point by calling for a "brisk" walk; yet studies have shown that walking has about half the caloric expenditure of slow running. Bounding up stairs or playing tennis or lifting weights strenuously for a few minutes are "anaerobic"—they force the body to run without oxygen for a brief period instead of requiring a continuous supply of air over an extended period. Aerobic exercise tends to develop slow-twitch muscles, whereas sprinters, for example, are not only born with a preponderance of fast-twitch muscles but continue to add to them with practice. It's true that the start-and-stop exercises associated with fast-twitch muscles cause fat to break down as they cause surges in blood to the muscles. But aerobic work accomplishes even more, simply because it's extended for longer periods of time.

The champions of walking point out that jogging has spawned a whole new industry of specialists in foot care. But injuries to the knees and feet are a small price to pay for a healthy heart, and such injuries are usually self-correcting. Ray Peat argues that women have special medical problems as a result of running: amenorrhea (the stopping of regular menstrual periods), varicose veins, and prolapsed uterus. Dr. Jane Ullyot has put these claims into perspective in her excellent books on exercise: the rumors appear to be greatly exaggerated. There is nothing inherently dangerous about missing periods—some women have even suggested running might be thought of as a form of birth control. Prolonged exercise can increase the risk of clotting, but this is easily overcome by sufficient intake of vitamin C. Some writers have warned against poor blood circulation and lactic acid buildup in the legs. Research at the University of California has recently questioned the long-standing theory that lactic acid is the cause of muscle fatigue: it now appears that it can be utilized as a fuel. And the general strengthening of the capillaries in aerobic exercise easily compensates for the alleged loss of circulation caused by jogging.

Dr. Peat advances an interesting theory on *how* to perform your exercise, whether you prefer running or walking: Do it with a happy face. He points to Russian studies that show that the brain, which "consumes a tremendous amount of fuel," is often overlooked in the exercise equation. "A walk through interesting and pleasant surroundings consumes more energy than does harder but more boring exercise." In any event, exercise should not be stressful. Trying to make your walking "brisk" can be quite stressful.

Now, the bonuses of aerobic exercise:

1. It appears to help the body use nutrients more efficiently.
2. It appears to be the only method of changing one's inherited metabolic "setpoint."

I have already mentioned, back in Chapter 2, how research into obesity has confirmed that each of us is born with a sort of thermostat that regulates when we start to burn fat. This is why some apparently overweight people fail to lose pounds even on a starvation diet. Women are especially the victims of a lack of understanding of this principle, both because of societal pressures on overweight women and because of the old prejudice, now happily changing, against women's exercising. They are discouraged from doing the only thing that can help them in severe overweight problems: aerobic exercise. For the same reason, overweight or obese women tend to overeat. Without adequate exercise, they metabolize nutrients poorly and so instinctively try to get more nutrients by eating more. Without exercise, they also fail to seek out those high-quality foods that the body craves in aerobic workouts: complex carbohydrates for fuel and high-quality protein for muscle rebuilding.

Dr. Gail Butterfield, assistant professor in the Department of Nutritional Sciences at the University of California, recently reported on her preliminary findings on how exercise can boost food values. Three groups of women, ranging from sedentary to highly active, were followed over a six-week period, and it appears that the most active had appreciably more vitamin C and iron in their bloodstreams on a diet similar to that of the sedentary. In other studies, vitamin B_6 and protein were metabolized better by those who did aerobic exercise than by those who did not.

As further investigations are made into the "set point" and the food-efficiency effect of exercise, we may find that these are far more than bonuses of aerobics. We may come full circle to discover that these are, in fact, the mechanisms behind the protective action of exercise against heart disease. We may find that the exercise of the heart muscle and the stimulation of the capillaries are secondary to the effect of exercise in delivering more nutrients to the arteries and in helping remove stores of fat.

A Personal Carbohydrate Plan for Your Personal Best

Ten years ago, when jogging was just beginning to become popular, a young woman came to me for psychiatric advice on the simple problem of how to stop smoking. Her family history made her high risk for heart disease, and her fiancé's quite realistic concern increased her desire to quit. She was willing to try hypnosis, mood conditioning, or any sort of psychological support. I noticed that her medical history showed that she was an active person, but apparently in the stop-and-go sports. I suggested an aerobic exercise program as a long-term solution, even though counseling seemed to be temporarily working. A friend of mine, a professor and a long-distance runner, had remarked to me casually that all his friends had stopped smoking when they took up running.

What I learned from this case was more interesting than a novel cure for smoking. This young woman also began to change her eating habits. It was to be expected that she would need more carbohydrates: they are the most readily available fuel. But she then reported that she was working more efficiently and had fewer mood swings—problems that she had not mentioned because all her friends seemed to have them, too. Could it be that adding complex carbohydrates to her diet was having a calming effect, contrary to what the theory of low-carbohydrate diets proclaims? Then I realized that *on balance* she was actually lowering her carbohydrate level; her exercise was accounting for more than she had added to her diet.

From this simple fact it seems probable that one explanation for the sense of self-esteem and well-being that runners report is that this sort of aerobic exercise is actually another form of carbohydrate regulation. Dr. Barbara Edelstein, in *The Woman Doctor's Diet for Women* (Prentice-Hall, 1977), writes, "Carbohydrates are the chief villain in the disease of overweight, because overweight women cannot tolerate them." Carbohydrates, she explains, can convert to fat instead of to energy when they're too prevalent in the diet; the concomitant rise in blood sugar can make women tired and depressed. Carbohydrate regulation is, of course, the first and major phase of the Listen to Your Body diet. We can see why, in the case of carbohydrate regulation by exercise, it is especially important to women. Women already have larger fat reserves, lose weight less easily than men, and are faced with a monthly cycle of metabolic changes that predispose them to mood changes. Stop-and-go exercise does not accomplish sufficient carbohydrate regulation to compensate for all of this on top of an intake high in carbohydrate.

I now regularly prescribe aerobic exercise—swimming, cycling, jogging—as a method of carbohydrate regulation. Exercise is more understandable in these terms than as a way of burning calories, or as a means of preventing heart disease. The connection between food and exercise is rapidly becoming more obvious. Exercise not only can control what and how much you eat, but how you make use of what you eat. And food can control how easily you exercise and what benefits you obtain from exercise.

Because of a lack of hard evidence, exercise physiologists have been unable to agree on the role of nutrients in exercise. It's clear that carbohydrates are the main fuel, but it would be a mistake to leap from this fact to recommending a high-carbohydrate diet for heavy exercisers. Recently, evidence has been accumulating to indicate that protein and several minerals and vitamins are critical for maximum athletic performance. Dr. Michael Colgan of Rockefeller University has tested marathon runners and found that the addition of a vitamin and mineral supplement to their training regimen significantly improved their performance. I have another way of approaching the subject. Let's put aside performance for a moment and consider the benefits of aerobic exercise mentioned throughout this chapter.

Endurance exercise is, first of all, something you must enjoy—otherwise it will be stressful and counterproductive. To be effective, it must not be a form of tension; it must be a form of relaxation. Deep breathing alone is a formidable way of relieving stress; you can practice it while you're driving, riding in a bus, or watching television. What foods or what eating patterns help promote these aspects of exercise?

First, get in the habit of taking plenty of liquids before as well as during prolonged exercise. A simple signal of whether you're getting enough liquids is the color of your urine: it should be light. Most of the disagreeable aspects of endurance exercise are caused by a lack of liquids *during* the exercise. You may not feel thirsty until you finish a long run; but then it's too late. You may unconsciously be saying to yourself, "Well, that wasn't much fun. I may not try that again."

Second, choose your liquids carefully to make them a regular source of key nutrients. Tomato juice is a good source of potassium, which is depleted in heavy exercise. Women especially need such minerals as zinc, iron, and magnesium, which can be obtained in meat or fish broths. Try to avoid tap water, which may contain fluorides as well as chlorine, in favor of mineral water or water that has been exposed to air for a while. Likewise avoid sweet juice drinks in large quantity; they may be rich in carbohydrates but they are the simple carbohydrates that are responsible for rapid changes in blood sugar.

Third, make sure you have adequate protein. Many of the aches and pains that discourage exercising are the result of muscle breakdown from lack of protein. Try to eat protein as the first meal of the day, because protein activates the metabolism and helps the body assimilate fat and carbohydrates more efficiently. It's also helpful to exercise early in the day, for this is when the adrenal hormones need to be stimulated. Since digestion "shuts down" during exercise, there's no reason to make your exercise unpleasant by working out on a full stomach. A logical pattern, then, is to jog, for example, first thing in the morning, and then have a light but hearty breakfast with good protein, such as eggs.

Fourth, choose foods that stimulate appetite-control hormones so that your exercise will also be a weight control program. The hormone cholecystokinin, or CCK, is a prominent control factor in satiety. There is no one specific food that stimulates the production of CCK, but in general protein, fats, and acid juices contribute to higher CCK. Because coffee and tea are acidic, some investigators have suggested these common beverages (along with diet drinks!) as a means of appetite control. But the caffeine in these drinks may also stimulate insulin production, which tends to excite the appetite. Exercise itself is a way of increasing CCK; this mechanism explains why heavy exercisers tend to lose their voracious appetites rather than become even hungrier after a workout. In short, cooperate with the good effects of your exercise program by concentrating on protein food sources, and at least some fats.

Fifth, choose your carbohydrates carefully and try to eat them first in a meal. Complex carbohydrates contain natural fiber, which promotes a longer digestion time and hence avoids rapid rising and falling of insulin levels. Also remember that vitamins C and E, which protect against the formation of free radicals, are not wasted if they wind up in the gut—as many critics of vitamin supplements argue. When complex carbohydrates are eaten first in a meal, they prepare the way for the absorption of fats, and so keep the fats out of storage.

Many people tell me that their aerobic exercise naturally directs them to foods and eating habits as exemplified in these five rules. There is no doubt that this is true—for some people. If two activities work well together, each will stimulate the other. But you can also consciously try to practice those good habits that contribute to successful exercise. There is no panacea in tricky food substitutions; there is no way to fool your body. The important thing to realize is that aerobic exercise has a purpose that is especially suited to women: a method of both mood and weight control quite unlike competitive athletics. And the foods that contribute to that purpose *must* be a high priority for women.

11
Change of Life
—for the Better

The goal of equality-before-the-law of the sexes is not furthered, in my opinion, by seeking *sameness* between men and women. We cannot disregard obvious differences in muscle mass, physical size, bone structure, hormones, and biochemistry between the sexes at every age. Differences in brain development and emotional capacities are more subtle and at least have little to do with legal rights. Although women are now entering the formerly male preserves of weight lifting, distance running, and, in general, blue-collar jobs, neither laws nor role-changes nor ideology can alter fundamental biological differences between the sexes. The capacity to bear offspring touches every part of a woman's life, whether that capacity is fulfilled or not. This basic difference presents real opportunities for women—if they use their difference instead of denying it. In Chapter 4 we looked at the menstrual cycle in some detail. Here let's take a look at menopause.

Change of life is a very specific thing for a woman: the end of her monthly cycle. It has overt metabolic consequences, such as the infamous "hot flushes" and other mild discomforts. This time of life signals the approach of "old age" and associated feelings of sexual decline and perhaps depression.

There is a great deal of psychological reaction that colors our understanding of menopause. Irritability and mood swings are often attributed to a woman's undergoing the one-to-two year period of change of life, when perhaps all we really see are the discomfort and embarrassment of flushes, sometimes the insomnia and fatigue that result from those flushes when they occur throughout the night. Psychiatric illness is now known to be *no more common* at the menopausal age—about 48 to 52, with a trend upward—than at other times. Dr. Myrna Weissman of the Yale University School of Medicine confirmed this in a study of depression and precipitating stresses among women between ages 45 and 55 and younger and older groups. Other research indicates only a slight increase in requests for psychiatric treatment at the menopausal age. Life stresses that are common in this period can be considered "midlife crises," and are similar for men and women: the maturation of the family, the diminution of enthusiasm for one's job, the questioning of one's sexual powers. But women suffer other, more specific problems directly related to hormonal changes, such as urinary tract infections, difficulty of sexual intercourse, and probably a tendency to obesity.

Our understanding and treatment of these problems, as well as of the problems of aging in general, are keyed in an obvious way to nutrition and nutrient therapy. For the brain is here the major factor in how we react to hormonal changes and in how those changes can be affected. As we learn more about that marvelous supercomputer that regulates every function of our body, we are beginning to find that drugs and medications are the enemy and that only through the body's own biochemicals can we hope to improve our brain functioning and thus our quality of life.

Start with the recently discovered fact that there is a chain of relations from the brain to the immune system to disease and malignancy. Several researchers have suggested, for example, that severe emotional stress can cause a breakdown in the immune system such that breast cancer will appear in women within six to eight months. One such researcher is Dr. Marian Diamond of the University of California at Berkeley. She is

currently looking for the mechanism between stress and malignancy, with emphasis on biofeedback as one possible preventive
measure. I have mentioned her work in brain research in Chapter 3; of interest in this chapter is the connection, which she has
shown in animal studies, between female hormones and the
cerebral cortex. "If we take the gonads out of the male at birth,"
she says, "and train him in our enriched environments, we
get the same changes as we do when the gonads are present.
Also, if we take the gonads out of the male at birth, we don't
change his right-left pattern. It stays the same. But if we take
the gonads out of the female at birth, her cortex grows bigger.
And we can change her right-left pattern if we take the ovaries
out."

In various animals, the right hemisphere of the brain is
thicker than the left *in males*. The right side controls visual and
spatial functions. Though the female brain has better balance in
size, her left hemisphere predominates to some extent: this is
the part of the brain that controls language. It has been argued
that the brain acts as a whole, so that this split-brain potential
does not mean that girls are necessarily better at language arts
and boys better at architecture or mathematics. But brain researchers have uncovered other differences between the male
and female cortex as well. They react to changes in the environment differently. Since hormones affect not only the lower
centers of the brain, but the vital cortex as well, it seems probable that the great changes that occur in women's hormones at
menopause have far-reaching effects on her health, sense of
well-being, and longevity.

We know that as far back as we have been able to gather
evidence, women have outlived men by several years. In spite of
high risks in childbirth in previous centuries, women have always been stronger against diseases of childhood and middle
age—and they have largely been spared in their youth the risks
of warfare. The invisible hand of evolution has somehow taken
these facts into account by providing for more births of boys—
even though the X and Y chromosomes of the sperm, which
respectively determine female or male, unaccountably seem to
be randomly dispersed. Just as hormonal imbalances may be at
the root of the far greater incidence of diabetes, osteoporosis,
and arthritis in women, this same biochemical change at the

change of life may also presage her ability to resist the "killer" diseases in men.

Because the male is able to father a child well beyond the age at which women stop menstruating, there is an underlying psychological affront to female sexuality at menopause. But it is only psychological. If a woman has remained sexually active up to this time of life, there is no reason why she can't maintain that interest through menopause and beyond. And the same nutritional standards that apply to fertility and potency at an earlier age also are critical now. This brings us, once again, to the subject of progesterone.

Estrogen therapy in menopause is a standard practice of physicians, even though it has been hotly debated in medical journals. The proponents of estrogen admit that breast cancer is a potential outcome of estrogen replacement. A recent editorial in the *Journal of the American Medical Association,* however, argues that "this low incidence of malignancy *must* be weighed against the anticipated gains from therapy." The authors cite alleviation not only of flushes, but of osteoporosis and atherosclerosis as well. "Estrogens rank among the safest of all pharmaceuticals," they state. "In more than 40 years, millions of women have been treated with presumed replacement doses of a large array of products; toxic reactions and side effects have been minimal."

The very fact that estrogen is here referred to as a "pharmaceutical" shows how drug-oriented medical thinking has become. The reality is that estrogen is one of many hormones whose interactions we are only on the threshold of understanding. What we do know is that in this "alphabet soup" of biochemicals, estrogen and progesterone are antagonists; and we have excellent evidence that it is progesterone that is the hormone that is out of balance in both menstruation and menopause. Further, there is ample evidence that the observed effects of estrogen in osteoporosis and atherosclerosis are illusory. In *The Biochemistry and Physiology of Bone* (1972), G. H. Bourne states that X-ray analysis does not show any restoration of bone mass; in fact, growth hormone stimulated by estrogen is known to aggravate the disease. Its proponents claim that estrogen results in less excretion of calcium in the urine—hence retention of calcium for the bones; but any toxin has this effect, and the calcium may be retained in the soft tissues. In the case of heart disease, it has been shown many times that estrogen causes a magnesium deficiency, which in turn promotes clotting.

As a naturally occurring biochemical, estrogen would not be expected to have serious side effects. Those that it has are no doubt the result of the drug formulations in which it is sold. In her recent textbook on endocrinology (the study of hormones), Constance Martin sums up the pluses and minuses this way: "Estrogens are not useful if administered over long periods of time." In my own practice, I have found progesterone, magnesium, vitamin B_6, zinc, and selenium to aid in the metabolism of calcium and produce remarkable reversal of serious osteoporosis. Since estrogen is known to inhibit brain-cell development, it seems highly unlikely that this hormone would have beneficial effects over an extended period of time.

Between the ages of forty and forty-nine, women who used oral contraceptives during their thirties risk heart attack at a rate two or three times greater than the risk for same-age women who never took the Pill. And if they currently take the Pill, their risk is four times greater. Smoking further increases these risks. In terms of total numbers, the danger of blood clots and stroke is even more severe in this group, since stroke is much more common than heart attacks among women this age to begin with. By emphasizing the same nutrients that protect women in premenstrual syndrome and menopause—especially those that are involved in progesterone synthesis (vitamins A, C, E, and pantothenic acid)—the risks of circulatory problems and heart attack are also minimized. Protein and the B vitamins, especially B_6, help regulate estrogen levels. An interesting side effect of vitamin E (side effects of nutrients are virtually always *beneficial* ones) is the slowing down of skin wrinkling. This antioxidant not only protects the heart against free radicals but also keeps the elastic fibers of skin supple, and for the same reason.

Aging: What We Talk About to Anyone but a Doctor

It's a common complaint that there are too few gerontologists. The common reason given for this is that no one wants to go to an "old age" specialist—until it's too late. Yet much could be done to improve the quality of life of people as they age, from menopause on, if only they knew how to ask their doctors the right questions.

In my psychiatric experience my most demanding geriatric case was an eighty-four-year-old woman who suffered from a severe depression at the time of the Suez crisis. Now, she was neither an Egyptologist, a shipping company magnate, nor a stockholder in an oil company. What happened was that this crisis precipitated our first energy crisis in this country: because ships couldn't get through the Suez Canal, we didn't have enough gasoline to go around. And apparently she despaired of being able to fuel her limousine—to see her lover of 45 years! And she was unable to walk because of a severe case of os-teoporosis that left her with painful hip joints. What a pity that she had allowed herself to be depleted of such minerals as calcium, magnesium, and phosphorus and probably vitamin D, which crippled her even as she had kept many other of the best things in life well in mind. It turned out that a psychological approach to her anxiety proved worthless; only by restoring her physical well-being was I able to reach her spirit—long after the oil was flowing again.

Linus Pauling made an interesting observation on the subject as far back as 1960. "There exists no reliable way of measuring the physiological age of an adult human being," he wrote. "The best way seems to be to look at him, and then to say how old he appears to be." Another way to look at it is quite hopeful: you are as old as you look.

I have always believed that accurate diagnosis is the critical factor in maintaining health. What should you test yourself for, then, as you begin to feel your age? A physical checkup in the best of clinics will give you a blood workup, urinalysis, and a multiple chemistry panel, prominent among which are choles-terol and uric acid measurements. In nutritional medicine this is not enough. Long before you begin to sense that you're not as spry as you used to be, it makes sense to have a complete bio assay of the major vitamin levels and a hair analysis of minerals. In suspect cases, the more expensive amino acid pathway analy-ses are the most advanced and clinically helpful tools modern medicine now has. When all these tests are done methodically and economically on a large scale, they will revolutionize the practice of preventive medicine, which I would define as the science of slowing the aging process.

Since diabetes figures so importantly in women over the age of fifty, there are several additional tests I routinely recommend to them. The simple glucose tolerance test remains a valuable procedure, not only to demonstrate the extent of hypoglycemia or diabetes, but also to educate the patient in the role of blood sugar in feeling well and in maintaining healthy blood vessels. We can now also measure the extent to which glucose is chemically bound to proteins of red blood cells. Because this condition is proportional to the average of blood sugar over a four month period, it gives us a longer view of how well a patient is metabolizing carbohydrate. As a result we can make more accurate predictions of potential damage to the proteins of blood vessels, nerves, kidneys, retinas, and the lenses of the eyes. At the same time, by measuring insulin tolerance we can be prepared to prevent such damage.

"Overutilization" is a fighting word in today's medical scene. It implies unending tests and extravagant procedures that physicians order only because they know an insurance company or a government program will pay for them. Thorough diagnosis, I firmly believe, more than pays for itself in the long run— even if most tests turn up nothing startling. In my experience, all the tests I have mentioned are far more productive than anything else done in an annual checkup. The real waste is the mindless prescription of drugs, often on the theory that if one doesn't work we'll try another. University of Maryland pharmacology professor Peter Lamy charges that physicians are especially thoughtless in dealing out prescriptions to the elderly:

> I once asked a group of physicians about a new prescription analgesic that had just come on the market. About 75 percent said they had already prescribed it. I asked them if any of them knew how much it cost. They said, "What do we need to know that for?"

What happens is that older patients ignore a medicine if it costs too much; they don't want to appear to be complainers. Lamy tells of a woman who stopped taking a hypertension medication.

When her doctor discovered her blood pressure remained high, he doubled the dose. The only thing that saved the woman's life was that she decided not to buy that, either.

We are now finding what we should have suspected long ago: drugs work differently in older people than in their juniors. Not only do people change metabolically throughout life—but as they get older they take more medications. According to the American Geriatrics Society, those over the age of sixty-five account for a third of the drugs we dispense. And the proliferation of drugs—many of the over-the-counter variety—has created a maze of problems because of their unpredictable interactions. Worse, the aged are stripped of vitamins and minerals as their metabolism breaks down and as drugs block the absorption of nutrients. Dr. Lamy says, "We expect old people to be dizzy, to be somewhat confused . . . when, indeed, it may be a vitamin deficiency induced by chronic drug use."

In my practice I have found that virtually every woman I would classify as physiologically old has had one or more serious deficiencies. After sufficient doses of nutrients to overcome these, each patient has been able to become essentially drug-free. This is not surprising when you consider a study done a few years ago by Dr. Alfredo Lopez, Professor of Medicine at Louisiana State Medical School. Together with dieticians Barbara Yates and Susan Jackson, Dr. Lopez examined 130 patients of a large university hospital, selected as a balanced sample. Approximately half of the patients suffered from some degree of protein malnutrition. He concluded, "It seems most physicians forget to think about a patient's nutritional status, which is so important in prognosis and treatment."

The management of diabetes in the United States has been similarly haphazard. Dr. Marvin Siperstein, Professor of Medicine at Veterans Administration Medical Center in San Francisco, notes that the standards established in the glucose tolerance test for diabetics failed to take into account the natural decline in the ability to metabolize sugar as people age. Millions of people were labeled diabetics and put on special programs ever since the American Diabetes Foundation set up their standards in the 1930s. "It was the grossest misdiagnosis," says Dr. Siperstein, "in medical history." The standard treatment for diabetes—a low-sugar, low-carbohydrate diet—has also been shown quite recently to be 180° off the mark. Several British studies have led the way in suggesting that a 50–60 percent carbohydrate share of the diet, especially if rich in complex carbohydrates and fiber, is the best approach.

I would also suggest that the role of nutrients in handling diabetes has been consistently underrated, under both the old and the new protocols of treatment. Complex carbohydrates and fiber contain just the vitamins and minerals that help the metabolism deal with sugar. Vitamin A is needed to synthesize the adrenal hormones, such as cortisone, which is the antagonist of insulin; in diabetes, a permanently high blood sugar level is poorly monitored by insulin. Vitamin C in high doses has been shown to cut the need of insulin doses in half. In insulin-dependent diabetics, blood glucose was lowered significantly by means of a high-fiber diet; but one of the main minerals in crude fiber, chromium, is known to be essential to the utilization of glucose. The B vitamins and magnesium are depleted in a high-sugar diet, so it is reasonable to conclude, as we will see, that a complete treatment program for diabetes must take many nutrients into account.

On top of everything else, our understanding of diabetes has been skewed all these years by the inclusion of supposed "prediabetics" in the statistics that have gone into our studies. When the standards by which diabetics were diagnosed were narrowed, Dr. Reubin Andres of the Gerontology Research Center in Baltimore said, "Think of it, several million people 'cured' by the stroke of a pen!"

Dr. Andres and others at the Center have campaigned for a more realistic understanding of aging in several other health areas: obesity, tuberculosis, pneumonia, sexuality, and malnutrition. The Center has conducted a longitudinal study of aging for more than 25 years, which may well be the first large-scale program for the total environmental approach to longevity. From this work we already know that overweight has been exaggerated as a medical concern for the aged. Lung tests have shown that smokers have a physiological age ten years older than their nonsmoking peers, but that virtually full recovery is possible after two years of giving up cigarettes.

Women and Meganutrition Will Have the Last Word

The longevity of women seems also to be matched by a better quality of life in those extra years. Why this is so may be answered for the same reasons in both cases.

Life expectancy in the United States, though lower than that of several European countries, is at an all-time high for both men and women—for both, it's in the seventies. Women still enjoy a four- to five-year edge. Yet we are clearly reaching a point of diminishing returns as the percentage improvement declines each year. A recent study of survival after heart attacks showed that in the decade from the mid-1960s to the mid-1970s there was virtually no improvement—despite huge outlays for research and much technological ballyhoo. An editorial in the *Journal of the American Medical Association* accompanying the report declaimed, "Such a conclusion is a bitter pill for those of us who have used and taken for granted the efficacy of improved medical care."

There are three factors in our diet and environment that stand out in clear relief as the reasons for this self-imposed limitation on human longevity:

1. The enormous and unprecedented pollution of the last 150 years, mainly caused by cigarette smoking and gasoline combustion.
2. The appearance of refined sugar and flour in the same period, alone accounting for a tenfold increase in sucrose over that supplied in natural foods.
3. The reduction in nutrients in the daily diet, chiefly vitamin C, because of methods of food manufacture and preparation as mankind has gone from a gathering to a growing to a purchasing society.

In all three cases, women have enjoyed something of a protective edge. Women are only now beginning to smoke like men and to enter the workplace where pollution from heavy metals and hydrocarbons is a way of life. Because of their greater susceptibility to "sugar diseases," such as diabetes, women in advanced years have had to watch their diets more carefully for unwanted sucrose. And the nutrient requirements of the menstrual cycle and childbirth have, when proper food was available, made women more conscious of nutrition. In a sense, women have been protected to some extent by their greater needs. What women can now teach the rest of the population is that to live longer and to live better longer are not just accidental products of that "invisible hand" of evolution.

Each year another wonder drug is announced as a possible solution to the problem of aging. In fact, many of these are not drugs at all, but nutrients. First there was choline—to improve brain functions, specifically memory. Then apomorphine and L-dopa—to normalize the neurotransmitter dopamine in the brain. Recently, attention has been focused on synthetically derived biochemicals, such as interferon—to counteract such diseases as cancer. Enzymes derived from soil bacteria have been proposed as a means of breaking the cross-linking of nucleic acid molecules. "Blood washing" to eliminate toxins has been suggested. All these treatments are expensive, some prohibitive; and they appear to be piecemeal solutions to fundamental problems.

The nutrient therapy approach is available now, is inexpensive, and goes to the heart of the problem. This therapy includes dealing with free radicals by means of the antioxidants, vitamins E and C, plus carotene, selenium, and cysteine. It includes the improvement in enzyme activity and the immune function through dietary adjustments of carbohydrates and emphasis on various trace elements. The nutritional approach to "turning back the clock" is so multifaceted and individualized that it may seem hopelessly intricate for self-care. Yet I think I can summarize a reasonable approach for any woman over the age of fifty:

- There are several nutrients that anyone over fifty often has trouble metabolizing, and that are also needed especially with advancing age to repair bone and tissue. Most of us can't rely on our diets to get enough, so we must take an extra amount in pill form. The RDAs for the two most important, calcium and magnesium, are respectively 800 and 300 milligrams for women over fifty. I suggest assuring yourself of this amount in a supplement alone.

- Vitamin C has numerous important benefits for older people, along with the other major antioxidant, vitamin E. Look for a supplement that supplies at least the RDA for E, and take extra C, up to 6 or 8 grams a day with meals. You will quickly discover how much you can tolerate without the "overdose" effect of diarrhea.
- Beyond the age of sixty-five, B_{12} and folic acid are especially difficult to absorb by mouth. But they can be injected intramuscularly. It's just good sense to ask your doctor for a shot of these two nutrients in the amount he or she feels necessary, twice a year, which would arrest any dangerous deficiency. Without these two B vitamins, cell growth and repair could not go on.
- Put your mind at ease about any mineral deficiencies by having your doctor order a hair test once every year or two. This is now a simple and inexpensive procedure, and is quite reliable when properly interpreted.
- As we have seen in detail, both the definition and treatment of diabetes are undergoing considerable changes. It is important to remember that while susceptibility to this condition is age-related, diabetes is not an inevitable part of growing old! Watch for signs of diabetes after the age of fifty: hunger, dizziness, irritability, nausea—the same indications of low blood sugar in hypoglycemia. If you have any reason to suspect diabetes, ask for a glycosylated hemoglobin test. Then be prepared to deal with diabetes on a nutritional basis—with a nutrient and fiber-rich diet, vitamins A and C, and extra chromium, magnesium, and the B vitamins. Only a nutritionally trained physician can prescribe the right program, at the right time, for you.
- The other most important test to watch is an annual serum cholesterol reading. Remember that the high-density lipoprotein measurement (HDL) shows how much of this *protective* form of cholesterol you have against heart disease.
- In addition to the Listen to Your Body diet as described in Chapter 2, there are several adjustments you can make in your eating habits to compensate for advancing years. As you grow older, your metabolic rate declines, so you need

fewer calories. Also, after the age of sixty-five your protein needs decline, so a higher proportion of your total calories can be in the form of carbohydrates. (There is no exact formula to ascertain your ideal protein intake; recall the study of hospital patients earlier in this chapter, half of whom were protein-deficient. Taper off, but don't go to extremes!) Since your bowels are more sluggish at this age, you may wish to add a simple bacteria to your diet—acidophilus culture—to keep regular and protect yourself against intestinal problems. This culture is available in any health foods store and in many milk products.

- For various reasons related to hormonal changes, women over fifty may experience depression, lack of concentration, or moodiness, more of which seems serious enough to warrant a doctor's care. Treat yourself first by varying your carbohydrates according to the Listen diet. Then follow up, if necessary, with a super B-complex supplement which contains 50 milligrams each of the B vitamins and 0.4 milligrams of folic acid. For most women, a dose of one to ten such tablets during the course of the day is quite effective. If you experience headache or nausea you simply reduce the dose as needed for comfort. The simplest remedies should always be tried first.

- It has been said again and again and I will repeat it here: no medicine can substitute for exercise. We tend to become increasingly sedentary as we age. Now that there are fewer societal pressures against being seen in our old clothes or shorts, running through the streets or cycling around town, there are few excuses to put off aerobic exercise. (In a recent study of the incidence of sudden death during heavy exercise, researchers concluded that precautionary stress tests were not justified by the risk. Don't delay getting started on a consistent exercise program.)

- The interactions of drugs are highly unpredictable. And individual drugs have variable effects on you over time and as you change. So be concerned about any non-food you put in your mouth. Don't be afraid to ask your physician about the purpose and effects of any drug he or she prescribes. If you feel you need another opinion, tell your doctor. Above all, tell him or her if you're not filling the prescriptions for any reason. If you don't have this degree of cooperation with your doctor, you should consider another one.

The contrast between drug treatment and nutrient therapy becomes sharper as we age. Our bodies become less resilient against the onslaught of drugs. Nutrients become more conspicuous by their absence! We have every reason to look to nutrition for making those years truly golden. And there is a larger lesson.

We know more about vitamins and minerals and their effects in the body than about any other aspect of medicine. We are also learning that antibiotic medicine is reaching a crisis point. Professor Marc Lappé of the University of California at Berkeley says, in his recent book, *Germs That Won't Die*, that "medical hubris" is threatening us with the indiscriminate use of antibiotics as more than 8 million pounds of them are added to animal feed to promote meat production. "The Age of the Miracle Drug is dead," he writes. "Only the most short-sighted observers could hope to reconstruct that wonderful era some forty years ago when we believed we were on the verge of chemically conquering all the infectious diseases. We tried, but the evolutionary prowess of the microbes won out."

It's time to go back to our roots.

12
Basic Questions Women Ask

The American woman—homemaker, careerist, student, or any combination of the three—is more inquisitive than her male counterpart concerning questions of health. And she is better informed. I have suggested that the reason for this lies in her sensitivity to her own fluctuations in well-being. She does, indeed, listen to her body.

I have discussed health questions with women on three levels: first, as a physician; second, as a lecturer and in other public appearances; and third, as the president of the Orthomolecular Medical Society. I have had the benefit of a broader forum, ranging from the very practical to the esoterically scientific. So I think I am in a position to answer the commonly asked questions with a better understanding of what women want to know—and with as much objectivity as it's possible for a single physician to have. As in any important field, there is considerable disagreement in the interplay of medicine and nutrition. In the following 12 questions and answers I will give the critics of my point of view equal time. I have confidence in the ability of the concerned woman to make up her own mind on the basis of "the whole truth."

1. What is your general rule for a healthy, long life?

Linus Pauling summed it up best in a paper he wrote some years ago in a scientific publication: "Avoid sucrose, take a fair amount of vitamins, stop smoking cigarettes, and you'll have a longer and happier life." He went on to give the major evidence for the role of large doses of vitamins in special cases: schizophrenia, arterial disease, surgery, and so forth. Dr. Pauling, of course, is not a medical doctor, and his great contribution to the field of medicine (carried out at the Linus Pauling Institute of Medicine and Science in Menlo Park, California) is in bringing the powerful analytical tools of biochemistry to the devising and interpretation of medical experiments. Since that paper was written, advances in all phases of nutritional medicine have been nothing less than startling. This is the "fine tuning" that we can now add to Dr. Pauling's basic prescription. As more and more controlled studies and clinical observations are reported in authoritative medical journals, it is becoming clear that nutrient therapy is the new direction of medicine.

I would add these general rules, based on what we now know of nutrition:

1. Avoid dietary extremes, including the "no-cholesterol" diet promoted by well-meaning officials and not so well-meaning manufacturers of foods.
2. Eat the best quality foods available, including those we have "junked" for the American dinner table.
3. Take a good vitamin-mineral supplement daily for the extra protection it gives you against disease.
4. Consider megadoses of the appropriate nutrients as the medicine of first choice when needed.
5. Exercise at least 30 minutes a day, three times a week.

Mega-nutrition is the *affordable,* natural key to a healthier, longer life.

2. The experts seem to disagree so often—what should I know about nutrition?

I agree that there is a lot of confusion in the media about nutrition. It's easy to seize upon a gimmick and try to turn it into a theory, and diet fads are often based on biochemical reactions that are quite real but relatively unimportant.

Here's a quick summary of all the biochemical information you'll need to understand mega-nutrition. There are at least six functions that any nutrient has in the body: (1) to provide structure, (2) to supply energy, (3) to regulate metabolism and hormonal functions, (4) to increase the rate of reactions, (5) to pass along genetic information, and (6) to supplement the nutrients the body can make from its own tissues. There are four major classes of biomolecules that carry out these functions: protein, fat, carbohydrate, and nucleic acids. In these classes are specific molecules that we commonly refer to by their chemical names—for example: insulin (a hormone, classed as a protein, that regulates blood sugar); retinol (vitamin A, classes as a fat or lipid, that "supplements" many other nutrients synthesized within the body); glucose (the chief carbohydrate in food, that supplies energy); and DNA (deoxyribonucleic acid, the nucleic acid responsible for hereditary characteristics). Some hormones are lipids, such as the female hormone estradiol, and some are proteins, such as insulin. Minerals are, of course, the basic elements that make up all organic substances—the chief ones being carbon, oxygen, and hydrogen. When these three are combined in simple structures that break down easily, as in sucrose, they form "simple" carbohydrates, as opposed to the complex structures of vegetables. The trace minerals usually *regulate* or *provide structure* as parts of protein. Energy is provided by carbohydrates, such as starch; by lipids, such as oils; or by the unique ATP, adenosine triphosphate, related to the nucleic acids. Amino acids are the building blocks of both protein and enzymes, though they differ in functions (in proteins to provide structure for hair, skin, bones; and in enzymes to act as catalysts for biochemical reactions). Protein is especially important because it cannot be derived from either carbohydrates or fats in the diet, whereas carbohydrates can, in effect, be derived from fats.

Biochemical reactions, in which complex molecules are broken down into simpler ones, are constantly going on in the body. This process is what we call a "metabolic pathway." One of the major advances in diagnostics in recent years is our ability to "look in on" the metabolic pathway of all 22 amino acids in a person's body, and so discover if any of these important nutrients are not being utilized properly.

I like my patients to understand as much about nutrition as possible, so that their programs make sense to them. This is, in a manner of speaking, the guiding motif of this book.

3. What about all the claims for vitamin C? Do they make sense?

It's natural to suspect an alleged cure-all. Indeed, I would be quite surprised if any medication or drug had more than a few unrelated benefits. But ascorbic acid is not a drug: it is a *nutrient*. And this makes all the difference in the world.

Nutrients have what might be called a "class action" effect. They potentiate biochemical reactions in many parts of the body at once, whereas a drug is designed to block or shut down a single or a few lines in the metabolic pathway. Linus Pauling has argued for the broad-scale potential of vitamin C on the basis of both clinical evidence and evolutionary data. Some day we may discover the precise mechanism of the action of vitamins, for example, that the antioxidant properties of ascorbate account for such diverse effects as protection against cancer and against the common cold. In the meantime, Pauling has made telling arguments to show that in our present evolutionary stage we are ascorbate-deficient animals. For example, it can be assumed that we generally eat what we need for survival; but in a vegetarian diet sufficient for survival we receive more than 50 times the ascorbate than the RDA. Therefore, that's the amount we probably need.

The critics of researchers like Pauling are not swayed by this type of reasoning, nor even by his evidence. Recently, a columnist in the *New York Times* blithely dismissed the thousands of reputable studies of vitamin C with this remark: "In truth, C may have real value beyond its ability to prevent scurvy, but the studies so far are inconclusive." The writer later mentioned studies of the effectiveness of ascorbate in the healing of wounds and burns, in asthma, in bone disorders, and several other areas. She failed to say why these studies were somehow "inconclusive" or indeed why she omitted dozens of other demonstrated benefits of ascorbate. As we have seen, subclinical deficiencies of vitamin C have been shown to be a cause of periodontal disease. The truth is that Pauling's extensive research into C and cancer and C and the common cold has yet to be successfully challenged.

Other nutrients, by the way, are showing similar panacea-like effects. Vitamin E, zinc, B_6, and the recently studied amino acid carnitine all have a remarkable number of benefits in apparently unrelated disorders or diseases. The critics are going to have to look at the research instead of dismissing any of these as a "cure-all."

4. Aren't there dangers in megadoses of some of the vitamins and minerals?

Yes, but they have been highly exaggerated. In the article mentioned above, the writers says, "C, like all drugs, has potential risks as well as possible benefits, and some people have become ill from taking a remedy that might actually be worthless for their conditions." This incredible bit of sophistry first equates ascorbate with a drug and then implies by the weakest connection that C is sometimes worthless and sometimes makes people sick!

The truth is that only two of the vitamins, A and D, have any serious liabilities for normal people, and only in huge doses.* There are two simple rules to follow for safety when dealing with vitamin and minerals pills: (1) Do not allow any candylike pill to get into the hands of young children; and (2) do not take extreme amounts of any substance for long periods without a doctor's advice, and watch for simple signs of overdose if you are treating yourself with large doses of any nutrient. There have been reports of headache with vitamin A and the B vitamins, and diarrhea or mild lethargy in the case of vitamin C. These reactions are easily stopped by cutting back on the dose. "Bowel tolerance," in fact, is one of the most convincing demonstrations of the effectiveness of ascorbate. When a person can tolerate huge doses of C (in the 60–80 gram range, as Dr. Robert Cathcart has shown in some cases of severe infections), it

* Warren D. Kumler, Ph.D., Professor of Chemistry and Pharmaceutical Chemistry Emeritus of the University of California School of Pharmacy, writes, "Except for vitamin E in individuals with rheumatic heart and specific individuals with rare diseases, most adults can take all vitamins in amounts several times the RDA without any toxic side effects."

is reasonable to assume that the C is needed by the body, and so isn't excreted.

Vitamins and minerals do have interactions; large doses of iron, for example, can block other nutrients. Nutrient therapy must be monitored carefully by a knowledgeable physician when specific disease states are being treated. One of the worst cases of anxiety I have ever seen was precipitated by eating a can of sardines—and I suggested it! A young woman had come to me after her psychiatrist had told her "You're just depressed." I recommended some foods to build up her nutritional status, but I didn't realize at the time that protein foods aged in cans or jars produce a substance called tyramines, which act like amphetamines. It was only after lengthy detective work that I pinpointed the cause of her attack—the sardines. This was perhaps the most dangerous reaction I have ever observed to any megadose of a nutrient, and it was solved simply by removing the offending food.

In the last analysis, nutrient therapy has two great things going for it: it's cheap and it's safe. It should not even be mentioned with drugs.

5. Does nutrition really have a place in the "killer" diseases?

The degenerative disease of cancer, atherosclerosis, diabetes, and arthritis is the scourge of our civilization. I say "disease" in the singular because they are probably all manifestations of a single chronic condition. That condition is *the general breakdown of the body's defenses, including the immune system.* And at the heart of the problem is the violation of basic nutritional practices, including protection from poisoning.

In cancer, Linus Pauling's research has been well publicized and typically misunderstood. Most recently, the nutritional armamentarium against cancer was summarized by Dr. Carl Pfeiffer and Dr. Eric Braverman, respectively of the Princeton Brain Bio Center and New York University School of Medicine. Reviewing the extensive literature on the subject, they recommend the following protocol for treatment of cancer

1. Vitamin C to tolerance, 10 to 20 grams a day.
2. Vitamin A at 50,000 units a day. ("These numbers look

large but remember that a dinner of calf's liver with carrots and beets will provide 25,000 u of vitamin A at a single sitting.")

3. Selenium in a dose of 100 micrograms in the morning and evening.

4. Vitamin E in doses of at least 400 units morning and evening. ("Some of our patients have taken 2,000 u AM and PM for years without any evidence of toxicity.")

5. Molybdenum at 500 micrograms a day.

6. Manganese gluconate, 50 milligrams morning and evening. (It is poorly absorbed from the gastrointestinal tract; if blood pressure is elevated in older patients from this large dose, substitute nuts and tropical fruits as the source for manganese.)

7. Zinc at 15 milligrams a day, or twice daily in severe cases.

Clearly, the control of cancer requires a complete program designed for the specific cancer and specific patient. There are many experimental treatments of various cancers, both here and abroad. Even laetrile has shown some success, and despite the negative test conducted by the National Cancer Institute this potent substance should not be ruled out when circumstances require extreme measures. The medical profession has a poor track record in its handling of cancer. Richard Bloch (cofounder of the tax-assistance firm with the simplified spelling, H & R Block Inc.) recently established a clinic at the University of Missouri in Kansas City, to give patients all over the country an alternative to any of the current treatments—a sort of second opinion from a broad review board. Asked why he declined to establish the center in a hospital, he cited the competition of doctors over their own institutions: "They like the prestige, the self-esteem, and the cash."

The program outlined above merely suggests the extensive part nutrient therapy has to play in cancer treatment. Research as well as clinical work is going on at an accelerated pace. A recent conference in Phoenix, Arizona, was devoted to progress in vitamin A treatment alone. In my own practice, I recall quite vividly how a person very close to me was spared the cauterization treatment of cancer of the cervix—vitamin A alone was successful. There are many cancers that are specifically female, so nutrient therapy offers women a great deal of hope where once they were defenseless.

In heart disease, diet is now well recognized as a crucial factor—but largely for the wrong reasons. As we have seen, cholesterol-phobia has been over promoted and the role of the antioxidant vitamins (C and E) and the collagen-building nutrients (C, zinc, etc.) has been slighted.

Any physician who treats diabetes and arthritis with insulin and aspirin alone, respectively, is not doing his or her job. Any drug, in fact, should be considered a last resort in these diet-related diseases. There are so many correlations between the diet and the disease, in both prevention and in treatment, that no one can ignore them any longer. If your doctor prescribes a drug without exploring nutrient therapy for any of the killer diseases, find another doctor.

6. Can I get all my nutrients in a balanced diet?

Yes—if you *can* get such a diet, and you are in good health. But our eating habits and our food supply have changed drastically, for the worse, in the last few generations. And when you are sick, most nutrients simply can't be supplied in sufficient dosage from food alone. How the food industry and organized medicine have fought against nutritional progress is an interesting story.

The food supply in the United States had been sufficiently tampered with by the turn of the century that the editor of a medical journal could write, in 1913:

> Away with the white loaf and the package breakfast food! Use whole wheat, the natural, unpolished brown rice, old-fashioned oatmeal and unbolted corn meal. Man may not live by bread alone but he can come mighty near it if he gets the real article. . . . Vegetables should not be boiled, but steamed. . . . Nuts are rich in proteins and fats and to a large extent they can take the place of meat. The same can be said of the legumes, which indeed are a perfect substitute for meat. . . . But even among physicians there is still a decided lack of appreciation of the importance of the nutritive salts in the human dietary.

Then in the next two decades the vitamin deficiency diseases—primarily pellagra and scurvy—became well understood and publicized. A new era in nutrition research seemed to be underway. As Robert Benowicz puts it:

> Between 1920 and 1950 enthusiasm for nutritional studies among scientists was at fever pitch. . . . Optimistic reports in the scientific literature brought a lavish expenditure of research time and money. Investigators—intent on discovering another group of wonder drugs equivalent to antibiotics and sulfanilamides—were, however, thwarted in their efforts to bend supplementary vitamins into therapeutic tools capable of curing such then dread diseases as polio.

Research funds now went into the search for drug cures for disease, and the pattern persists to this day. Some 10 *billion* dollars have been spent on cancer research since the war on cancer was announced. We continue to refine the cut-burn-poison approach, unwilling to face the fact that the chronic degenerative diseases have resisted all attempts at cures—in the real sense of the word—with these surgical, radiation, and chemical therapies.

By the mid-70s, however, a trickle of funding and interest appeared for nutritional medicine. Largely because of the prestige of Dr. Linus Pauling, Dr. Roger Williams, and a handful of others at major medical schools, nutrition studies began to be taken more seriously. Research that had been washed overboard in the enthusiasm for drug studies was rescued. Adelle Davis was at last recognized for what she was: a popularizer with two great scientific strengths—inquisitiveness and practical experience. The obvious interest of consumers in nutrition—as evidenced by the boom in health food stores, cooperatives, and vitamin sales—began to make an impact on the medical and food-processing fraternity. Cereal manufacturers took note of the antisugar feeling of parents by creating whole-grain and sugarless products. It can't be denied, of course, that some processors tried to capitalize on this new interest in honest foods by distorting the meaning of "organic" or "natural" products. But a ground swell of public demand for less adulterated, more wholesome foods could not be ignored even by General Mills. Finally, at a time when the major medical associations and societies of nutritionists were still reassuring us that we were getting healthier on the American diet, the United States Senate issued, in mid-1977, an explosive report on the downward trend of our nutrition. Entitled "Diet Related to Killer Diseases," this was the first official recognition that things were hardly getting better and better in every way.

The evidence had been there all the time, but now, in one official volume, one could read:

- The niacin versus schizophrenia report by Osmond and Hoffer, the review of a nine-year study, in *Lancet,* 1962.
- The work of Carl Pfeiffer, using hair analyses, on zinc deficiencies and copper excess in schizophrenics, reported in the *International Review of Neurobiology* and the *Journal of Applied Nutrition,* in 1972 and 1973.
- The first controlled study showing the effectiveness of megavitamin therapy (C, B_3, B_6) in schizophrenia, by Linus Pauling and others, in 1973.
- A double-blind crossover study by Rimland, Callaway, and Dreyfus on the effect of B_6 on autistic children, 1974.
- The Feingold study on the effects of food additives and salicylates on hyperactive children, 1974.

In short, the Senate Committee on Nutrition and Human Needs heard not only about the deterioration of the nation's food supply as the result of processing, but about the use of nutrients to cope with the diseases of subclinical malnutrition. And the participants in these hearings were not representatives of health food stores, but scientists from such institutions as the University of California, Massachusetts Institute of Technology, and the University of Rochester School of Medicine.

Finally, a report financed by the Department of Agriculture, the "HANES Report," dispelled the idea that vitamins are amply supplied in the American diet. For example, vitamin A deficiency enough to cause *symptoms* of visual deterioration (pre-night-blindness) was found in 40 percent of the population of the country, projected from samples in the survey.

"Balanced diet" is a death sentence for millions of Americans who are able to survive while the symptoms of the chronic diseases go unnoticed. When their bodies start breaking down and diagnosable maladies show up, it's usually too late. Their lives are shortened by subclinical malnutrition just as if they had been taken down a chemically poisoned mine shaft.

7. Isn't there a lot of quackery in the health food industry? The general press is full of sensational stories about the "health food rip-off." Many of the critics of nutrient therapy hold respected positions in federal agencies and at leading universities. So it's important to give this issue a thorough airing.

The *National Enquirer* is a publication that routinely announces miracle health potions on the slimmest evidence. Recently, this supermarket journal of fad and gossip quoted several prominent medical men on the subject of health foods and megavitamins. Their verdict: "nutritional quackery" that costs Americans $3 billion a year.

Dr. Frederick Stare, a professor of nutrition at Harvard University School of Public Health, had this to say: "Taking megavitamins is like eating dirt. It certainly isn't going to help you—and it might very well hurt you. If you want to know what the dollar rip-off on it is, it's virtually every penny spent." The chairman of the National Academy of Science's committee on dietary allowances, which establishes the RDAs, confirmed this opinion: "By far the largest proportion, perhaps even 99 percent, of every dollar spent in this country on megavitamins is a waste." These are serious charges.

First of all, I would answer that any person who bandies such charges in a tabloid that reaches millions of people should be prepared to answer for the sickness and death he or she might cause by suck reckless remarks. Most people who take vitamins do not take "megavitamins." Supplements of various vitamins and minerals are the common purchase.

But how did we get to such a state in this country, after all we know, that to be a "health nut" is thought deviant behavior, and to treat yourself with diet is considered bizarre? The American Medical Association, in fact, has recently issued warnings against those who offer nutritional medicine, and the word "quack" is being used rather freely these days to describe anyone who thinks that foods can in some cases work better against disease than drugs.

One of the most tireless and vociferous critics of nutritional medicine, Dr. Victor Herbert of the Bronx Veterans Administration Medical Center, recently published his views in *Nutrition Cultism* (Stickley, 1980). The dust jacket proclaims that this book "gives 16 tips on how to spot food quacks . . . and legal resources for victims of nutrition fraud." In a chapter excoriating "the vitamin craze," Dr. Herbert takes particular aim at the members of the medical society of which I am recent past president:

> A popular cult exists around the use of megadoses of vitamins to treat a host of disorders, mental and physical. Megavitamin therapy and orthomolecular psychiatry are largely supported by anecdotal accounts (testimonials) which are worthless as scientific or legal evidence. . . . There are many false but popular misconceptions about vitamins, particularly among "health food" users. The majority of the charismatic "nutrition" preachers to the public promote these misconceptions in their lucrative books, magazines, and media appearances. . . . 21% of the general public and 37% of confirmed health food users erroneously believed that many diseases, including arthritis and cancer, are partly caused by lack of vitamins and minerals.

Nor does Dr. Herbert flinch at naming names. He begins his book with the following assessment of the work of Adelle Davis and Dr. Linus Pauling:

> Do you believe Adelle Davis' suggestions that if you follow her nutrition advice, you won't get cancer? Did you know that Adelle Davis died of cancer. . . .
> Do you believe Linus Pauling's claims that megadoses of vitamin C prevent colds and cancer? Did you know that Prof. Pauling gets colds, as do we all, as reporters at one of his New York news conferences observed firsthand. . . .

Venturing into specifics, Dr. Herbert proceeds in the same introduction to take on two subjects popularized in recent books on weight loss and hyperactivity in children:

> Until Einstein's equation, $E = mc^2$ . . . which may also be written (Calories = weight times the speed of light squared) is repealed, the only way to lose weight will be to eat each day less calories than you burn up. . . .
> The best evidence is that the claims that eliminating sugar, carbohydrates, and/or additives from the diet corrects behavior disorders and hyperactivity in children are based on coincidence rather than cause and effect. . . . The changes in

behavior are induced by behavior modification, and not by changes in diet content.

Herbert is an extreme case, but consider how the subject of vitamin supplements is treated day in, day out, in the press. One begins to get the feeling that vitamin supplementation is as "bad" as megavitamins. Some samples from recent popular books:

> . . . One concept which we must keep in mind throughout the discussion is that a healthy person who eats a well-balanced diet receives adequate amounts of vitamins from his food and, therefore, does *not* need any vitamin supplements. (Arthur S. Verdesca, M.D., *Live, Work and Be Healthy*, Van Nostrand Reinhold, 1980)

> The average healthy American adult consuming a typical balanced and varied diet requires no vitamin supplements. . . . Excess vitamin consumption serves no purpose except to risk serious side effects. (Herbert M. Dean, M.D., and John J. Massarelli, M.D., *Look To Your Health*, Van Nostrand Reinhold, 1980)

> The money (consumers) spend on vitamin and mineral supplements is, for the most part, wasted.
> When the poor consumer sees "RDA" on a label . . . he can be sure of one thing. . . . That the Recommended Daily Allowance recommends much more than he really needs. (David Reuben, M.D., *Everything You Always Wanted to Know About Nutrition*, Simon & Schuster, 1978)

On a recent talk show in San Francisco, the head of the Nutrition Department at the University of California referred to vitamin pills as a gimmick and advised listeners to reach first for a glass of orange juice.

Contrary to Dr. Victor Herbert, the general public that suspected a diet problem in such chronic diseases as arthritis and cancer were not being misled by "quacks." The medical fraternity will, I feel, eventually respond to lay people who want to know more about the effect of vitamins and minerals on disease. Meanwhile, the public is being pushed and pulled on all sides. The temptation of critics is always to look for the "rip off" behind every popular cause, and, indeed, American business has capitalized on the public's interest in nutrition. We see advertisements in the leading national magazines for "Myadec. If you want more." (Parke-Davis). Geritol tells us to "put back the vitamins your day takes away," with their Mega-Vitamins. There's Unicap T—"For up-tempo people." A. H. Robins tells us that "being active can drain a man's body of zinc—a metal more precious than gold for good health." Hoffman LaRoche takes a broad, statesmanlike position in advertising vitamins—for it is the leading manufacturer of ascorbic acid; whereas a smaller company buttonholes us, "Every heart beat depends on potassium. Are you short on it?" Nathan Pritikin touts his Longevity Center with the headline, "The joy of surmounting heart disease." And advertisements by General Nutrition Centers boggle the mind with such items as fertile eggs, low-sodium cornflakes, kelp, lecithin, and Super B-4 ("America's most wanted formulation!"). On the other hand, most books on women's medical problems contain virtually nothing about vitamins and minerals. Jane Brody's otherwise excellent compendium on nutrition contains two paragraphs on vitamins and relegates vitamin K to a line on a chart.

How can one know which way to turn? Dr. Roger Mazlen, chairman of the AMA's Council on Nutrition and Cardiovascular Disease, said in 1980:

> There is thus a paradox present, inasmuch as 75 years of great scientific advancements in nutrition and medicine were accompanied by a progressive decline in our dietary composition, and a progressive increase in our burden of chronic disease. The importance of understanding this paradox is critical from the stanpoint of both morbidity and mortality figures, and the financial aspect. The answers offer hope of salvaging and extending human lives and of reducing the awesome burden of disease.

Dr. Michael Sporn, chief of the laboratory of chemoprevention at the National Institutes of Health, says concerning cancer: "I continue to believe that a single multivitamin capsule is the best investment in health in America." In these two statements I see the best advice for a confused public.

Now, how about the charge of quackery? Dr. Joseph Beasley, Bard Center Fellow in Health and Nutrition, gives a penetrating overview of the issue: "Rarely does quackery arise where established medicine is treating a problem effectively." Yes, there is quackery, in and out of the medical profession. But name-calling on a level of the Big Lie has no place in a scientific endeavor. The worst nutrition in America exists, perhaps, in the main arena of medicine, the hospital. Here the graduates of our nutrition departments of medical schools serve twice-steamed vegetables and "convenience" entrees that would embarrass a second-rate restaurant. I have seen patients on restricted carbohydrate diets given orange juice between meals, and all-lettuce salads passed off as "green vegetables." Ray Peat, a biochemist who publishes a fascinating news letter about the frontiers of nutrition, tells this story about the prevalent view of "registered dieticians":

> A friend of mine who visited the Oregon State University nutrition department told me that a display there included books by Adelle Davis, Roger Williams, and Linus Pauling, in a display on "nutritional quacks." Adelle Davis had a degree in dietetics and nutrition from the University of California at Berkeley, and a master's degree in biochemistry from the University of Southern California School of Medicine. Williams, a professor in biochemistry (and the only biochemist to have been chosen as president of the American Chemical Society) has done research in nutrition for over fifty years, and is the discoverer of the B vitamin pantothenic acid, as well as having done research on other B vitamins. Pauling, Nobel laureate in chemistry (as well as in peace), created much of the scientific foundation for modern medicine, physiological chemistry, and nutrition. Maybe somebody is trying to glorify quackery by associating these people with the word!

Fortunately, the scientific literature on the role of vitamins and minerals is growing at a prodigious pace. No authority on nutrition has the right to ignore the equally voluminous record of clinical evidence for nutrients. Some epidemiologists have estimated that 80 percent of the population is deficient in magnesium, zinc, chromium, and selenium! Women are especially vulnerable to deficiencies in our society because their diet is generally more restricted both in variety and in total intake, even though they have potentially better access to more nutritious food.

If prescription drugs were subjected to the same critique for efficacy, safety, and cost as are nutrients, then we would truly hear cries of "fraud."

8. Do we really have hard evidence on deficiencies and specific nutrients?

For a doctor or any scientifically oriented person this is critical. So it was encouraging to see that the *Journal of the American Medical Association* published a report in late 1981 that acknowledged the existence of a "subclinical deficiency." Every physician who bases his or her knowledge of nutrition on the remembrance of a professor's words that deficiency diseases are rare in America should heed this study:

> Vitamin C deprivation in industrialized societies has seldom been severe enough to be clinically evident. . . . Recent studies supported by the National Institute of Dental Research now offer the first concrete evidence that subclinical vitamin C deficiency significantly increases susceptibility to periodontal disease. . . . The findings described here, together with previously established evidence, indicate several mechanisms by which vitamin C may aid the body in defending itself against periodontal disease.

Then, a definitive review of "the essential trace elements" appeared in *Science*, authored by Walter Mertz, director of a nutrition center of the Department of Agriculture. Essential elements were defined as:

1. Those that are needed to prevent impairment of optimal or suboptimal functioning.
2. Those that would, by themselves, restore such functioning if ingested in the right amounts.
3. *And* those that have demonstrated both of the above in more than one animal species, in studies by more than one investigator.

By these criteria, writes Mertz, these trace elements are now considered essential in animals (and human beings): silicon, vanadium, chromium, manganese, iron, cobalt, nickel, copper, zinc, arsenic, selenium, molybdenum, and iodine. Fluorine and tin should join these 13 when current studies are reported. (It's well known that fluorine is protective against tooth decay.) Consider: these minerals have been called "trace" elements because their concentrations are so small in the human body that originally we had no easy way of measuring them. They are the "mineral salts" that the medical journal called to our attention in 1913 (see Question No. 6). These are some of the deficiency signs of the 13 minerals listed above, in respective order, as identified thus far in animal studies:

Silicon: Growth depression, bone deformities

Vanadium: Growth depression, change of lipid metabolism, impairment of reproduction

Chromium: Relative insulin resistance

Manganese: Growth depression, bone deformities, b-cell degeneration

Iron; Cobalt: Anemia, growth retardation

Nickel: Growth depression, anemia, changes in liver, impaired reproduction

Copper: Anemia, rupture of large vessels

Zinc: Failure to eat, severe growth depression, skin lesions, sexual immaturity

Arsenic: Impairment of growth and reproduction, sudden heart death

Selenium: Muscle degeneration, pancreas atrophy

Molybdenum: Growth depression, reproduction difficulties

Iodine: Goiter, depression of thyroid function

In humans, we don't yet know for sure what symptoms are the unique result of deficiencies of these trace elements: silicon, vanadium, manganese, nickel, arsenic, and molybdenum. But the symptoms resulting from a lack of the other seven (not to mention fluorine and tin) are roughly the same as those in animals.

The role of selenium and silicon in aging has been well documented, and we are now able to make pretty good guesses about the functions of all the trace elements. As Mertz sums up the case:

> In the developed, industrialized societies, the exposure of humans to trace elements from diet and environment has changed during this century, and the change can be expected

to continue. Furthermore, many of our chronic diseases of major public health importance are of unknown or of suspected multifactorial origin, and theories on their etiology are open to new ideas that might involve any of the new trace elements.

So it's clear that mega-nutrition is far more complex than the idea of popping a multivitamin supplement, or of loading up on vitamin C when you have a cold. In addition to vitamins and minerals, these are some of the elements of our metabolism that must be taken into account in a complete medico-nutritional picture:

- Amino acids
- Essential fatty acids
- Fiber, in various forms of cellulose
- Enzymes and their hormonal interactions
- Antibodies and the immune system, antigens
- Chelation therapy and the interactions of minerals and vitamins
- Artificial and natural light
- Air and water pollution, ionization

In addition, various therapies not fully accepted in conventional medicine should not be neglected: dialysis, plasmapharesis, exercise therapy in relation to diet, thermal therapy, phototherapy, electrotherapy, acupuncture, massage, hypnosis, biofeedback, and various psychological therapies such as mood conditioning.

At this point you might be tempted to ask, Isn't this all lumped together as "holistic" medicine? My answer is that, broadly speaking, holistic physicians or practitioners consider themselves *outside* the mainstream of medicine, or at least as practicing an alternative to conventional medicine. I do not think this of mega-nutrition. All of the therapies and objects of study listed above are logical extensions of the long, scientific tradition of medical practice. For medicine has always asked only one question: How can I know more about my patient?

9. Aren't nutritional claims based mainly on anecdotes?
Clinical observations have always been denigrated as "anecdotal" or "testimonial." In current medical research, there is a

strong preference for the so-called "double-blind" or "double-blind crossover" study. The purpose of such studies is to remove any element of the placebo effect—"wishing it were so"—on the part of either the patient or researcher conducting the testing. Hence, "double-blind." In a "crossover," the group receiving the chemically inert pill—the placebo—later receives the drug or nutrient, and vice-versa, and the results are analyzed to further refine conclusions.

It is obviously not important to eliminate a placebo effect in cases where the benefit is so apparent that "wishing could never make it so." The pain of arthritis is a good example; but when even the patient finds it difficult to tell if he is in pain or not it is important to have adequate numbers of patients in both the control and the study group in a fully "blind" test. And statistical interpretation now becomes critical.

Nutritional claims are indeed based mainly on clinical observations. But then so are many of the advances in all areas of medicine. We don't even know how aspirin and the important heart medication digitalis work at the molecular level. There are no controlled studies of many of their known benefits. In a major article on chemical contamination in the *Journal of the American Medical Association* in 1981, Robert W. Miller begins: "Virtually every known human carcinogen and teratogen has first been recognized by an alert clinician." By examining the history of successful treatment of chemically contaminated individuals, he shows that there is a great value in "asking the patient what may have caused his illness." This story of his is typical:

> In 1977, several men engaged in the manufacture of dibromochloropropane (DBCP) wanted to have children, but their wives did not become pregnant. The men thought their work exposures were responsible. Their physicians thought not. Five of the men took semen specimens to a local laboratory, which declined to send the results to them, but agreed to send the information to a nearby university scientist, who was a consultant both to the union and to the company involved. He quickly confirmed the abnormal findings. . . . The workers not only suspected that the chemical in their workplace caused their sterility, but they also initiated the laboratory study to prove it.

In every doctor's work, there is a sort of informal protocol that is far more convincing than a small percentage increase in a double-blind study. This is what might be called the "light switch" effect. If you use a nutrient (or drug) and the problem goes away, then remove the treatment and the problem returns, you have discovered something rather basic. If you then repeat the "study" with various patients with the same result, you have discovered something rather important. One does not have to understand electricity to appreciate the effect of the "on" and the "off."

There are two things that need to be said about studies versus practice: (1) where the placebo effect is a big factor, the treatment is probably only of marginal value, and (2) no matter how many studies are known to the physician, it is mainly clinical observations that show the *relative* importance of various treatments. Advances are being made so rapidly in nutrient therapy, with such obvious success, that it is almost a fetish to insist on double-blind protocols to test them. Nevertheless, this laborious work is now being undertaken around the world and is being reported in the leading medical journals.

10. Is genetic engineering a part of nutrient therapy?
Much attention has been focused on the substances that occur naturally in the body and that can now be synthesized in the test tube, so to speak. Interferon, the natural antagonist of cancer, is a good example. Dr. Benjamin Siegel and his wife Dr. Jane Morton have done extensive work on this and other immunological effects. They ask the simple question: "If it is known that vitamin C in large doses produces significant increases in interferon in the body, why all the fuss about producing interferon synthetically at a tremendous cost?"

I should add that research on the benefits of interferon isn't airtight. But the point is this: American medicine will proceed on a drug-model even if a nutrient-model is readily available. The responsibility of any corporation is to maximize profit, and this applies equally to drug companies. Two controversial "drugs" make this point clear: DMSO and EDTA. I have mentioned both briefly in Chapter 1. Over the past 20 years dimethyl sulfoxide (DMSO) has been shown to be a powerful antiinflammatory agent with numerous medical benefits. Because it is so easy to manufacture, as a by-product of the timber industry, and because, as a basic chemical it is unpatentable, no drug company can afford to risk the hundreds of thousands of dollars necessary to secure FDA approval for general use. It has been approved for certain rare diseases where virtually nothing else works. As most people know, it is sold as a solvent in hardware and sports stores, but no one is deceived—people use it for all sorts of aches and pains, including arthritis. The chelating agent EDTA exhibits another "profit barrier" in medicine. Any mild acid, including ascorbic acid or vitamin C, will combine with certain minerals in the body and they will be excreted. The acid EDTA is designed to combine with the mineral deposits in arteries that are so badly blocked that they would otherwise require bypass surgery. EDTA has proved exceptionally effective in carefully monitored studies. It is not only much less expensive than surgery, but much safer, as well, especially for the elderly. Why is it not recognized for this use by the FDA? Again, because crisis-intervention medicine has discouraged any technique or drug that is an economic threat to itself. In short, the profit motive hinders objective medical research.

Genetic engineering is a way of making natural substances—nutrients or molecules normally present in the human body—into drugs. It has yet to be seen whether the effort in this new area of research will benefit medicine as much as a similar effort in nutrition.

11. How important is exercise in the nutrient therapy program?

For women it is perhaps even more important than for men. This is because exercise seems to have more of a hormonal effect than we ever suspected. It is well established, for example, that heavy exercise, such as running, can cause amenorrhea—the missing of a menstrual period or periods. When fat levels in a woman go below about 18 percent of total body composition, menarche may be delayed. The catecholamines released during heavy exercise have a beneficial effect on common depression—a frequent episode in the menstrual and maternal cycle of women.

It is important to see that exercise is not a cause of fatigue. After prolonged jogging, for example, one may be tired or even bone-weary; fatigue is something else. It is, in fact, the most frequent complaint I receive, and I presume it is the same for other physicians. As I stressed in Chaper 10, women who learn to exercise for at least 30 minutes in the morning, three days a week at a minimum, have more energy during the day. They work better, eat more wisely, and sleep effortlessly. Needless to say, they also find that they have at least 30 minutes of peace and quiet.

12. Are recipes a part of mega-nutrition?

I suppose I would seem to be remiss if I did not include a recipe section at the end of a diet book. Yet, what is a recipe? In the best sense, it is a way of preparing food nutritiously. In another good sense, it is a principle of food combinations. In the least important sense, it is a method of making processed food look better than it is. To use this book effectively, you don't need more than the general principles I can summarize here.

Consider the fact that most vegetables require cooking to be palatable (and this especially applies to grains, potatoes, beans). Yet we know that nutrients are preserved best if cooking can be avoided. This says something about the virtue of finding your right level of carbohydrates. Most carbohydrates are in those foods that require cooking, and most people eat too many carbohydrates.

Mega-nutrition means increasing your nutritional intake to the maximum. It means (1) cooking as little as possible, (2) including nutrient-rich foods in your diet (the "junked foods"), and (3) avoiding manufactured foods wherever possible. It means insisting on fresh vegetables at a restaurant. It means using the salad bar at fast food eateries. It means *thinking* about what you put in your mouth.

Yes, recipes are part of mega-nutrition. The basic recipe is simply *become food conscious*. In sickness and in health, think first of those things that *nurture* you instead of drugs that debilitate you. To a woman, this is second nature.

APPENDIX I

Suggested Additional Reading

Joseph Beasley: *The Impact of Nutrition on the Health of Americans.* Ford Foundation Report, 1981.
Jeffrey Bland: *Your Health Under Siege.* Stephen Greene Press, 1981.
George M. Briggs and Doris H. Calloway: *Nutrition and Physical Fitness.* W. B. Saunders, 1979.
I. J. T. Davies: *Clinical Significance of the Essential Biological Metals.* Charles C Thomas, 1972.
Ross Hume Hall: *Food for Nought.* Harper & Row, 1974.

Ewan Cameron and Linus Pauling: *Cancer and Vitamin C.* Linus Pauling Institute of Science and Medicine, 1979.
Isobel W. Jennings: Vitamins in Endocrine Metabolism. Charles C Thomas, 1970.
Betty Kamen and Si Kamen: *Total Nutrition During Pregnancy.* Appleton Century Crofts, 1981.
Roman J. Kutsky: *Handbook of Vitamins and Hormones.* Van Nostrand Reinhold, 1973.
Patricia McEntire: *Mommy I'm Hungry.* Cougar Books, 1982.
Lynda Madaras and Jane Patterson: *Womancare.* Avon, 1981.
Carl C. Pfeiffer: *Mental and Elemental Nutrients.* Keats, 1975.
June Roth: Cooking for Your Hyperactive Child. Contemporary Books, 1977.
Henry A. Schroeder: *The Trace Elements and Man.* Devin-Adair, 1973.

APPENDIX II

Recommended Daily Dietary Allowances (RDAs)

This list of nutrients is derived from that of the Food and Nutrition Board of the National Research Council, as revised in 1980. The RDAs are intended merely as guidelines, since they cannot take into account all individual biochemical variations (see Chapter 1). For example, though the government tables adjust requirements according to sex, weight, height, and age, women of the same weight, height, and age may actually have quite different nutrient requirements. To further complicate matters, when percentages of an RDA are shown on a food label, they are based on the 1968 RDAs. Finally, the *sources* of various nutrients affect their potency; for example, pure folacin can be four times as effective as the same dose in dietary form.

In spite of all these qualifications, this list can be helpful in evaluating your diet and in highlighting the special requirements of women at various stages of life. Since most people do not like to read tables, I have simplified the data to emphasize what is of greatest interest to the readers of this book. To make a realistic assessment of any deficiencies you may be developing, you should carefully list all the foods you have eaten over a typical week, noting approximate portions and cooking methods for each. This information can then be analyzed by computer. (See Appendix III for suggestions as to how to obtain this and other services.)

Nutrient	Women, Age 23–50	Pregnant	Lactating
Vitamin A, micrograms	800	1,000	1,200
Vitamin D, micrograms	5	10	10
Vitamin E, micrograms	8	10	11
Vitamin C, milligrams	60	80	100
Folacin, micrograms	400	800	500
Niacin, milligrams	13	15	18
Riboflavin, milligrams	1.2	1.5	1.7
Thiamin, milligrams	1.0	1.4	1.5
Vitamin B_6, milligrams	2.0	2.6	2.5
Vitamin B_{12}, micrograms	3.0	4.0	4.0
Calcium, milligrams	800	1,200	1,200
Phosphorous, milligrams	800	1,200	1,200
Iodine, micrograms	150	175	200
Iron, milligrams	18	18*	18**
Magnesium, milligrams	300	450	450
Zinc, milligrams	15	20	25

* Increased need in excess of usual dietary intake; supplements of 30–60 mg recommended.
** Continue supplementation for two to three months after delivery, then resume non-pregnancy level of intake.

Women age 19–22 have a requirement of 7.5 micrograms of vitamin D and slightly greater amounts of niacin, riboflavin, and thiamin. Women over the age of 50, conversely, require slightly less niacin and riboflavin and considerably less iron. The chief additional requirement of women under 19 is 50 percent additional calcium and phosphorus. Men's requirements are generally higher except for iron. Nutrients not shown here do not yet have an established RDA and are assumed to be present if these vitamins and minerals are adequate. In Canada, guidelines are generally higher for both men and women.

APPENDIX III

Diagnostic Services and Referrals

Several important diagnostic tools have been mentioned in this book: vitamin and mineral assay, hair test for trace mineral deficiencies, and computerized diet survey. Your physician may not be aware of or may not employ such services in his or her practice. If you wish to make use of them or if you need help in locating a nutritionally oriented physician, please write me at the address below. Enclose a stamped, self-addressed business-size envelope (#10) and the following information:

1. Your name and full address
2. The subject or specialty you are interested in (you may use the chapters in this book to identify the subject)
3. Your age and occupation, or the age and occupation of the person for whom you are requesting further information
4. Your reaction to the "Listen to Your Body" diet, in terms of weight loss, improved sense of well-being, or correction of a medical problem.

This information will help me in my research. In return, I will do my best to refer you to a nutritionally minded physician in your area who can order the diagnostic services you may require, or provide medical care as necessary.

Richard A. Kunin, M.D.
2698 Pacific Avenue
San Francisco, California 94115

Index

Acne, 55
Adenosine triphosphate (ATP), 86
Aerobic exercise:
  benefits of, 49–50
  carbohydrate regulation through,
    151–154
  forms of, 146
  general rules of, 147
  time period for, 146–147
  walking *vs* running, 148–149
  for women, 148
Aggression, junk food and, 116
Aging:
  diabetes and, 162–163, 166
  drug treatment in, 161–162, 165,
    167–168
  health maintenance and, 159–161
  nutrient therapy approach to, 162,
    165–168
Alcohol, 74, 75
  beer and wine, 131–132
  physical damage from, 130–131
Alcoholism:
  biochemical origins of, 133–134
  depression and, 131
  and food allergy, 136–139
  nutrient therapy for, 132–136, 139–
    142
  precursor of, 129–130
  in women, 128–129
Amenorrhea, 149, 189
American Heart Association (AHA), on
  cholesterol, 123–124

Amino acids, 50–51, 78, 171
Amniocentesis, 104
Andres, Reubin, 163
Animal fats, 19
Arsenic, 185
Arteriosclerosis, cholesterol and, 123–
  124, 125
Ascorbic acid (*See* Vitamin C)
Aspirin, 56, 65
Asthma, Vitamin B_{12} in, 10–11, 12
Atherosclerosis, estrogen and, 158–159
Atkins, Robert, 32
Atkins diet, 33
ATP (*See* Adenosine triphosphate)
Autism, birth-weight in, 103

Baking soda, for teeth care, 47
Bassler, Tom, 30
Beans, 106
Beasley, Joseph, 93–94, 182–183
Beauty:
  cosmetics and, 41, 42–43
  general health in, 41–42
  (*See also* Nutritional beauty care)
Beer, 131–132
Benowicz, Robert, 57, 177
Beverly Hills diet, 31, 32
BHC, 122
Birth control pill (*See* Pill)
Birth-weight:
  maternal diet and, 92–93
  neuropsychiatric disorders and, 103–
    104

Eggs, 60, 106
  yolks, 52, 55
Estrogen:
  in sexual dysfunction, 85
  for skin care, 53
  therapy, 72, 158–159
  in menstrual problems, 63
Evening primrose oil, 141–142
Exercise:
  benefits of, 143, 189–190
  caloric expenditure and, 36–37
  for elderly, 167
  food cravings and, 30
  role of nutrients in, 152–154
  safe levels of, 145–146
  (See also Aerobic exercise)
Eye problems, nutrients for, 47

Fast food, vs junk food, 116
Fasting, benefits of, 88–89
Fat is a Feminist Issue (Ohrbach), 88
Fats:
  deficiency in, 32–33, 74
  dietary adjustment of, 19, 22
Fertility problems (See Infertility)
Fetus:
  brain development of, 104–105
  external influences on, 105
Flynn, Margaret, 125
Folic acid, 12, 51, 166
  and B_{12} deficiency, 96
  deficiency of, 66
  during pregnancy, 96–97
  sexuality and, 83–84
Food(s):
  cravings, 28, 29–30, 37
  nutrient content of, 27, 176–178
  pesticides in, 122
  selection and preparation of, 13, 190
    cholesterol and, 122–126
    of cola alternatives, 113–114
    ethnic, 121
    fresh vs frozen, 112
    of junk food, 115–116
    for maximum nutrient value, 120–121
    natural flavorings in, 113
    nutrient-sparing, 112–113
    of processed foods, 117–121
    from scratch, 113

shelf shopping and, 111–112
  (See also specific foods)
Food allergy, alcoholism and, 136–139
Framingham study, 123
Fructose diet, 31
Fruit, daily amounts of, 114
Fruit juice, 113–114

Garlic, 121
Germs That Won't Die (Lappe), 168
Glutamic acid, in alcoholism treatment, 135–136
Glutathione, 11
Goiter problems, 85
Grains, 106
Gums, nutrients for, 47, 48

Hair problems, nutrients for, 46–47, 51–52, 56
Hair test, 52
Halogen displacement law, 47–48
HANES Report, 178
HCP (Hexachlorophene), 58–59
Heart disease, 77
  cholesterol and, 123–124, 125–126
  estrogen therapy and, 159
  milk and, 118–119
Heptachlor, 122
Herbert, Victor, 179–180
Herpes, 76–78
Hexachlorophene (HCP), 58–59
Histamine level, orgasm and, 83–84
Holistic medicine, 1, 186
Horrobin, David F., 140
Hydrogen peroxide, for teeth care, 47
Hyperactivity, and diet, 116, 180–181
Hysterectomies, unjustified, 8, 70

Infant mortality, 91
Infants (see Newborns)
Infertility:
  lead levels and, 101
  pollution and, 100
Iodine, 11, 78, 185
  deficiency of, 85–86
  food sources for, 48
  in teeth care, 47–48
Iron, 185
  absorption of, 107
  deficiency of, 48

197

Iron (*cont.*):
during pregnancy, 99–100
IUD, 85, 101

Jacobson, Michael, 124
Jarvis, D. C., 47–48
Jenner, Edward, 77
Junk food diet, effects of, 115–116

Lactic acid, 149
Lamb, Lawrence, 118
Lamy, Peter, 161
Lappe, Frances Moore, 121, 122
Lappe, Marc, 168
Laurel's Kitchen, 13
Lead, acceptable levels of, 101
Light shock, 47
Lindane, 122
Linoleic acid, 33, 75
Liquid protein diet, 2
Listen to Your Body diet, 15–39
body response and, 20, 23, 37–38
carbohydrate adjustment in, 17–18, 21
in crises, 38–39
fat and protein adjustment in, 18–19, 22
preliminaries to, 30–31
Longevity:
limitation on, 164
nutrition rules for, 170
of women, 157, 164–165
Lonsdale, Derrick, 116
Lopez, Alfredo, 162
Lysine, 78

Madaras, Lynda, 7, 63, 69
Magnesium, 85, 86
Male Practice: How Doctors Manipulate Women (Mendelsohn), 7–8, 71
Manganese, 185
Margarine, 114–115
Martin, Constance, 159
Massarelli, John J., 181
Mayer, Jean, 26–27
Mazel, Judy, 31, 32
Mazlen, Roger, 182
Medical profession:
anecdotal reports to, 72–73
and cancer treatment, 175

drug model in, 188–189
drug prescription practices of, 161–162
overutilization by, 161
and prenatal care, 91–93
women and, 7–8, 69–71
Medical research:
acceptance of, 77
profit motive in, 189
Megadose, 45
criticism of, 179–184
reactions to, 173–174
Mega-nutrition (*See* Nutrient therapy)
Mendelsohn, Robert, 7–8, 71
Menopause:
estrogen therapy in, 158
hormonal changes at, 156, 157
psychiatric illness and, 156
sexuality at, 158
Menstrual cycle problems, 63
nutritional deficiencies in, 65–66
Mertz, Walter, 184
Metabolic pathway, 171
Metabolic rate (BMR), exercise and, 36–37
Migraine headaches, vitamin C against, 64, 65
Milk:
allergies and intolerance to, 118
moderate intake of, 119, 126–127
pasteurization effects on, 117–119
in prenatal diet, 106
skim, 119
Miller, Robert W., 187
Molybdenum, 185
Morton, Jane, 188
Morton's Lite Salt, 113
Mouth problems, nutrient deficiency in, 48–49

National Enquirer, 179
Newborns, low birthweight in, 92–93, 103–104
Niacin (*See* Vitamin B_3)
Nickel, 185
Night blindness, 47
Nutrients:
deficiency in, 43–46, 184–185
druglike actions of, 9–11

Vegetarianism:
  protein deficiency and, 34–35
  vitamin B_{12} deficiency in, 96
  vitamin supplements in, 10
  zinc deficiency and, 107–108
Verdesca, Arthur, S., 181
Vitamin A, 51, 85, 163, 171, 173
  deficiency, 40, 47, 178
  for depression, 68
  in pregnancy, 99
Vitamin B, 116
Vitamin B_2 (riboflavin), 10, 47, 126
Vitamin B_3 (niacin), 10
  deficiency, 48
  skin reaction to, 55–56
Vitamin B_6 (pyridoxine), 10, 52, 159
  deficiency, 65
  in fertility, 86
Vitamin B_{12}, 10–11, 12, 96, 166
Vitamin C, 12, 85, 149, 154, 163, 173–174
  deficiency, 184
  for elderly, 166
  for herpes, 78
  for migraine headaches, 64, 65
  studies of, 172–173
  in teeth care, 57–58
Vitamin D, 173
Vitamin E, 11, 154
  deficiency, 40
  for herpes, 78
  overdose, 49–50
  in sexual capacity, 85, 86
  in skin care, 159
Vitamin K, 49, 50
Vitamin-mineral supplements, 13–14
  for alcoholism, 132–133
  for athletic performance, 152
  with contraception, 101
  criticism of, 181
  for elderly, 165–166

  megadoses of, 173–174, 180
  in pregnancy, 96–97
  for skin care, 55–56

Walking, in aerobic exercise, 148–149
Weight charts, revision of, 25
Weight loss:
  calorie intake and, 35–37
  and exercise, 149–150, 151–154
  metabolic rate and, 36
  societal pressure for, 24–25
  (*See also* Diet)
Weissman, Myrna, 156
What Every Pregnant Woman Should Know (Brewer), 92, 93
White, Philip L., 32
Williams, Roger J., 132–134, 135, 136
Wine, 131–132
Womancare (Madaras and Patterson), 7
Woman Doctor's Diet for Women (Edelstein), 151
Women:
  alcoholism in, 128–129
  body fat on, 144
  brain function in, 157
  disease incidence for, 8
  longevity of, 157, 164–165
  and medical profession, 7–8, 69–71
  nutritional requirements of, 5, 6
  physiological reactions in, 62–63
  prescription drugs and, 129
Wright, Jonathan, 10
Wurtman, Richard J., 81

Yaruyra-Tobias, Jose, 116

Zinc, 51, 185
  in sexuality, 7, 85
  in skin disorders, 55, 57
  sources of, 51
  soy effects on, 107

Titles of Related Interest from PLUME